Fresh Faced Makeup

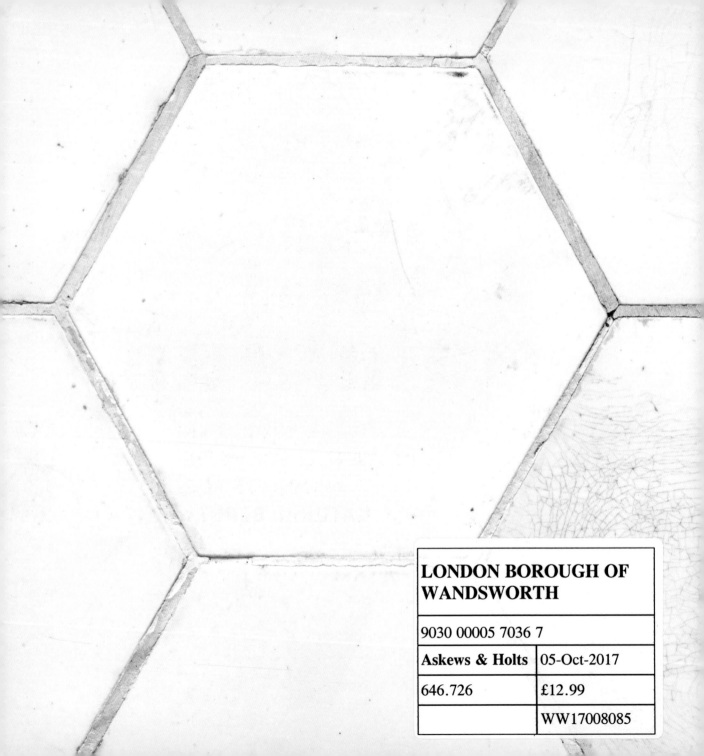

Alex Brennan

Fresh Faced Makeup

MAKE YOUR OWN SKINCARE & COSMETIC PRODUCTS FOR NATURAL BEAUTY

PAVILION

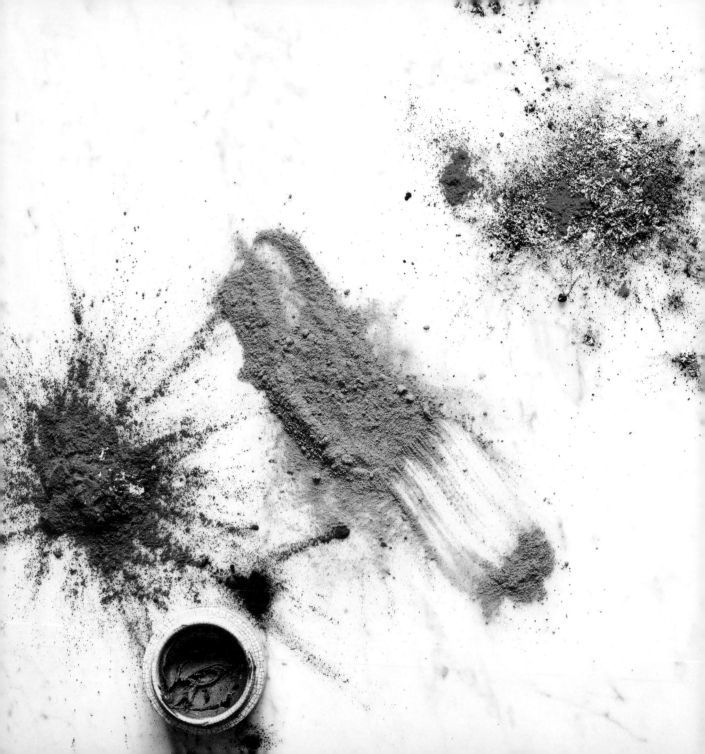

Recipe Menu

A Love Letter

Let me tell you a story... Four years ago, amidst a series of hugely stressful events and when I was trying to make a name for myself in the modelling world, all my hair started falling out. Stress can do unexpected things to the body, and it's not uncommon for cells to go on strike. But a model with no hair isn't something you see every day.

After a dozen doctor's visits and specialist appointments, I was disheartened and depressed; everyone could tell me what was wrong (alopecia), but not how to fix it. When all hope seemed lost, a dear friend suggested I look at the ingredients in my shampoo. Isopropyl alcohol, propylene glycol, sodium lauryl sulphate... holy moly! I mean, this was hazmat-suit stuff. What the hell were these ingredients and had I really put them on my scalp day after day?

In the end I took matters into my own hands and, armed with bottles of homemade shampoo and conditioner, my hair finally grew back. Then I started to really look at the state of the rest of my body – problematic skin, allergies, cellulite. Simple, one-ingredient, healthy alternatives – bought in supermarkets and health-food stores – have changed not just the quality of my skin but also my overall health.

Fast forward to today and I'm still outraged that nothing has changed in the beauty industry. Sure, we've got the organic movement flooding the airwaves but have you had a look at the ingredients in those products? Many of them are as aggressive as their non-organic counterparts, not to mention being murder on your wallet! My products offer sweet relief and now even friends who are makeup artists and models use them at home and on the job.

Learning and practising natural skin care has been amazingly beneficial and super EASY! If I can do it; you can do it. It's as simple as that! That first bottle of homemade shampoo changed my life and now I want to share with you all the little tips and tricks that I've discovered along the way. This book is for anyone and everyone who wants to make a change, and I'm so honoured to teach you everything I know.

Lots of love,

Alex Brennan

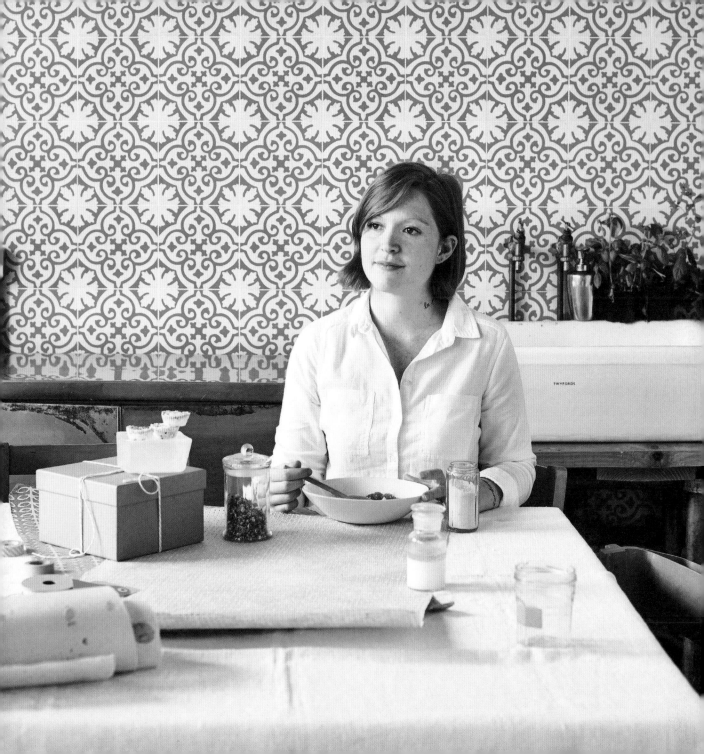

Getting Started

Most of the women I know – and most of the men, too – spend a lot of time grooming. It's a primeval, perfectly natural pastime (just spend some time watching primates). However, over time, as the cosmetics industry has grown and brought in billions of dollars for companies all over the world, the products we use for our grooming have become increasingly less natural.

The products you keep in your beauty bag are as individual as your likes and dislikes in life. This book is dedicated to all those special little concoctions that no bathroom, no dressing table, and no makeup pouch is complete without. Some are 'essentials'; others are just for fun. Most of these DIYs are quick to make, but if you want something that takes a second, just follow my #everyonelovesaquickie advice.

If you do a lot of travelling, then you'll know there's nothing better than your own shower (and your own bed), and while I'm usually fine with cleaning (and sleeping) in unfamiliar places, I never can get used to the impersonal atmosphere of a hotel room. Nothing reminds you you're away from home quite like the idea that someone else (someone you don't know, no less) has used the bathroom, looked in the mirror, slept in the bed. Whenever I find myself somewhere new, the first thing I do is unpack all my own little beauty products and place them on the dressing table and around the bathroom, then I run the shower (or the bath if they have one) and add a few drops of my favourite essential oil (ylang ylang) to the water. Instantly, I feel more at home.

If you're on the road and don't want to take a mountain of products with you, then I recommend packing a cleanser, toner and moisturizer (take a look at the #everyonelovesaquickie pages at the start of each section for ideas for the most efficient packing possible), a face powder, eyeliner and some all-natural lipstick – you'll find all these products and more in this book. I've split the book into beauty-specific sections – from looking after your face (with its really delicate skin, which is exposed to all sorts every day), to correcting pimples and then soothing and smoothing out blemishes. Then, I've given you recipes for eyes and lips, nails and perfume, to complete the makeup arsenal. Everything here is easy to make and totally natural to use – after all, you are naturally beautiful.

'Learn with your mind, listen with your body'

Four years ago, when my awakening began, a dear friend taught me the value of listening as well as learning. Anyone who's ever been on a diet knows that you have to learn to ignore your own desires – your body is hungry but you pretend you can't hear it; it's not your tummy grumbling, it must be an echo. Learning to ignore my own thoughts, feelings and impulses was how I ended up in a terrible mess.

If you'd asked me back then what was 'wrong' with me, I could've rattled off a list of carefully studied diagnoses I'd been given; I could even have told you all the ways to 'cure' them; but if you'd asked me how I was feeling, there'd have been silence. I wasn't oblivious to my emotions, I just plain didn't want to acknowledge them – sometimes pain does funny things to people.

Part of removing all the questionable chemicals in my house and testing a bunch of recipes was learning how to listen. How could I know my body was not okay if I never gave it a chance to tell me?

In this magical era, where we hustle and bustle day in, day out and human contact comes in the form of texts, emails and Instagram feeds, I think we are all a little guilty of neglecting ourselves. Ever thought to yourself, 'I just don't have the time'? There's a reason readymade everything is available, whether it's pre-packaged, drive-through, home delivery or ordered online; trust me, I get it, but it's also the reason suppliers never have to change their products. Humans are busy, ergo they'll keep buying what they don't have time to make. Let's get this straight, I'm not one of those knit-your-own-breakfast types with too much time on my hands – I'm drawn to convenience as much as anybody else. When I started creating products, I made a shampoo and a conditioner and that was it. For six months I carried on using all the other regular rubbish I'd been buying for as long as I can remember. But, the ongoing task of listening to my body meant I eventually had no choice but to throw that stuff away and go back to basics. I could feel something wasn't right and even though my hair had begun to grow back (in great condition, I might add), my skin was a mess, I had cellulite, I was tired all the time and I was developing allergies left, right and centre.

I pulled all the beauty and cosmetic products out of my cupboards and laid them on the floor of my living room (a little excessive perhaps but hey, that's me). I had a notepad and pen next to me and carefully wrote down every ingredient I didn't know, had never heard of, or just plain sounded dodgy. It took hours!

When I'd finally compiled my list I sat down at the computer – okay, in truth I took a nap, watched a couple of DVDs and chilled out – but when all of that was done, I set to work and between me and Google I had a fair description of each ingredient. On my last ingredient – DBP – I stumbled upon a website called the Skin Deep Database (www.ewg.org/skindeep), a comprehensive list of every chemical (organic and traditional) ever used in cosmetics, skin care and perfumes. Talk about hitting the jackpot – this was everything I was looking for and more…

The Terrible 'Touch-me-nots'

Also known as the 'dirty dozen', this is a glossary of AVOIDS in beauty products. (Quick warning – this is going to read a little like a science lecture as these ingredients are specialized chemicals.)

Every day we use products that we think are ok; but in truth most are not proven to be safe, and manufacturers don't have to tell us so. Neither the EU or the FDA (Food and Drug Administration) require pre-market approval of beauty and cosmetic products and ingredients, so products could be marketed without government approval, regardless of what tests show. There are 25,000 chemicals used in cosmetics and most have not been tested for long-term effects.

Who knew?! I know I didn't until my own health was affected. It's best to always read the labels and know what's in your products. Don't be scared… just get educated and avoid the baddies on the list below.

BHA & BHT
Used as preservatives, there are concerns that these are toxic to organs and cause irritation to the skin, eyes and lungs. BHA has been linked to endocrine disruption.

Coal Tar Derivatives
Many synthetic colours are derived from coal tar and are potentially carcinogenic. Look out for p-phenylenediamine – used in numerous hair dyes - and colours with the prefix D&C or FD&C.

DEA, MEA & TEA
Keep an eye out for any ingredients that include the acronyms DEA, MEA and TEA (diethanolamine, monoethanolamine and triethanolamine respectively). These are used as surfactants and they carry many health concerns and can increase the risk for cancer.

Dibutyl Phthalate (DBP)
Used as a plasticizer, fragrance ingredient and solvent, this acts as an endocrine disrupter and can damage the reproductive system.

Formaldehyde
This carcinogen can be released by several different preservatives used in the cosmetics industry. Low-level use of these ingredients is permitted but in the EU a product containing over 0.05 per cent formaldehyde must carry the warning 'contains formaldehyde' on the label.

Parabens
This family of preservatives has gained a lot of negative publicity in recent years and rightly so; they mimic oestrogen and can disrupt the endocrine system that regulates our hormones.

Parfum/Fragrance
This term can refer to any mixture of synthetic fragrances which don't have to be named individually. They are associated with allergic reactions, asthma and respiratory problems.

PEGs
AKA polyethylene glycols, these are derived from petroleum and are used in many skin cream bases. Impurities such as 1,4-dioxane, found in may PEG compounds, have been linked to cancer.

Petrolatum
Obtained from petroleum and used in some hair products for shine and as a moisture barrier in some lip products and moisturizers. Associated with organ system toxicity; contamination concerns.

Siloxanes
Any ingredient ending in '-siloxane' or '-methicone'. Used in a variety of cosmetics to soften and moisten. There are various concerns around endocrine disruption and organ toxicity.

Sodium Laureth/Lauryl Sulphate (SLES/SLS)
These foaming agents have been known to cause irritation to the skin, eyes and lungs. They may be contaminated with ethylene oxide and 1,4-dioxane, which may increase the risk for cancer.

Triclosan
A preservative and anti-bacterial agent that is found in toothpastes, cleansers and antiperspirants. Irritating to the skin and eyes and suspected of hormone disruption.

The Ins & Outs of the Organic Movement

'I couldn't find anything on the market free of harmful ingredients so I decided to create my own.'
Heard this before? It is, of course, the line used by every 'organic' skincare or cosmetics brand that comes along. The organic movement isn't all bad – it's definitely a step in the right direction – but what if I told you that just because an ingredient comes from the Earth it doesn't make it healthy? Shocked? So was I! Now, I'm a huge fan of Mother Nature and what she offers, but not everything growing is meant for us. This is why I get a little red-faced when talking about organic product companies as I tend to find they use ingredients that no one really looks into, and then slap a massive price tag on. Let me show you what I mean. Meet the top four 'organic' beauty ingredients...

Cetearyl Alcohol

What it's used for Emulsifier, emollient, foam booster, stabilizer, thickener.

Avoid it because Possible eye, lung and skin irritant.

What it's made from Originally derived from sperm-whale oil, but now comes from palm oil.

Alex weighs in A long time ago I ordered a bucket of cetearyl alcohol to experiment with. When it was heated it smelled absolutely horrendous. The warning labels were a bit off-putting, too: 'Do not get in contact with skin', 'Do not get in contact with eyes', 'Do not breathe dust.' So... a product that's usually in lotions shouldn't be in contact with skin? Yes, it gets diluted, but wouldn't you rather use a moisturizer that has ingredients you don't have to worry about?

Propylene Glycol

What it's used for Thickener, filler.

Avoid it because It has just about every side effect: the risk of cancer, reproductive toxicity, usage restrictions, allergies and immune system toxicity, skin and eye irritations, organ system toxicity, endocrine disruption and neurotoxicity. It is also a penetration enhancer, meaning it penetrates skin cells, getting right into the bloodstream, carrying other chemicals with it.

What it's made from Derived from glycerine.

Alex weighs in If you're using a supposedly 'natural' deodorant, odds are it contains propylene glycol. Many of the natural companies sell 'paraben-free' and 'aluminium-free' deodorants, but they still contain propylene glycol because it's a cheap ingredient that makes a clear and thick deodorant bar.

Tocopheryl Acetate

What it's used for Antioxidant agent, labelling appeal (it is often listed as Vitamin E Acetate).

Avoid it because Certain studies suggest that it's toxic on skin and other organs. The biggest concern is that it can be contaminated in the manufacturing process by hydroquinone, a chemical that is highly toxic and carcinogenic in high concentrations.

What it's made from Made by combining natural vitamin E with acetic acid.

Alex weighs in 'Now with vitamin E!' sounds great on a label. This form of vitamin E has a longer shelf life and it's cheaper than natural vitamin E which is why companies use it. What they're not telling you is that it has risks for contamination and that it's a skin irritant and toxin. Some companies even try to pass this nasty chemical off as a 'natural' ingredient.

Limonene & Linalool

These little fellows are in every organic product under the sun. Limonene is a colourless liquid hydrocarbon derived from citrus peels and linalool is an alcohol found in flowers and spice plants. Sound ok? Well...

Limonene is believed to disrupt the body's ability to regulate serotonin and dopamine (the happy hormones), and so may be linked to depression and anxiety. Linalool breaks down when mixed with oxygen, forming a toxic by-product that can cause skin disorders, stress and brain malfunction.

The Harmful, the Organic & the Natural Alternatives

Below is a list of every necessary ingredient in cosmetics and skin care; the harmful, the organic (yep, still harmful) and the all-natural substitute. Next time you're swayed to buy the organic product or if you already have a shelf-full take a closer look and see how many contain these naughties.

Unfortunately, the word 'natural' has little meaning when it comes to cosmetics labelling, which is why it's important to know what all the ingredients on the label are so you can make an informed decision about what you're putting on your skin. Remember, ingredients are listed from highest percentage to lowest.

COLOURS OR COLOURANTS

Coal-tar derived colours in cosmetics are a concern because coal tar is a carcinogen. Some colour additives are not approved for food products, but may be added to cosmetics such as lipstick, which are inevitably ingested.

Look out for (and avoid):
Aluminum lakes, astaxanthin, azulene, canthaxanthin, sodium copper chlorophyllin (chlorophyll), D&C / FD&C colours, p-phenylenediamine, ultramarine.

Natural alternatives?
The above are used in many so-called 'natural' and 'organic' products so always read the ingredients list. True natural alternatives include beet powder, annatto, henna and caramel. Mica powders and iron oxides also have natural components and are non-toxic and non-irritating.

EMOLLIENTS

Emollients prevent moisture loss. Some synthetic emollients do not allow the skin to breathe and can actually cause it to become irritated and dehydrated.

Look out for (and avoid):
Acetylated lanolin alcohol, butyl adipate, capric/caprylic triglyceride, ceteareth, cetearyl alcohol, cetyl esters, cetyl palmitate, coconut fatty acids, cyclomethicone, decyl oleate, dicaprylate-dicapriate, dimethicone, disodium, cocoamphodiacetate, dodecatrienol, eucerin (petroleum jelly), glycerol-mono-stearate-palmitate, glyceryl cocoate, glyceryl stearate, hydrated palm glycerides, hydrogenated oils, isobutyl stearate, isopropyl lanolate, isopropyl myristate, isostearyl-isostearate, lauryl lactate, octyl palmitate, octyldodecanol, oleth-2, paraffin, petrolatum, squalane, stearate, stearyl alcohol.

Natural alternatives?
Plant oils such as almond oil, avocado oil, coconut oil, hazelnut oil, jojoba oil, olive oil, safflower oil, sesame oil, sunflower oil and tamanu oil. Shea butter, cocoa butter and beeswax are also natural emollients.

HUMECTANTS

Many synthetic humectants (to soften skin) draw moisture from the lower layers of skin but fail to replace it, giving softer skin in the short term, but drying it out over time.

Look out for (and avoid):
Butylene glycol, ethylene / diethylene glycol, PEG compounds (e.g. polyethylene glycol), polypropylene glycol, propylene glycol.

Natural alternatives?
Natural humectants deliver moisture to the lower levels of skin while also attracting moisture to the surface. Aloe, lecithin and vegetable glycerine are among them.

EMULSIFIERS
Emulsifiers suspend tiny drops of oil in water (in creams and lotions) or water within oil (used in heavier creams). They are often derived from petrochemical gases.

Look out for (and avoid):
Acetylated lanolin alcohol, alkyl polyglycoside, cetearyl alcohol, betaine, carbomer, carboxymethyl cellulose, cocamidopropyl betaine (coco betaine), ethyl acetate, ethylene glycol distearate, fatty acid alkanolamide, glyceryl mono-di-oleate, glycerol mono-di-stearate, PEG-100 stearate, PEG-25 hydrogenated castor oil, polysorbate, sodium lauryl sulphate, sodium sulfosuccinates, sorbitan esters, sorbitan stearate, stearyl alcohol, triethanolamine (TEA).

Natural alternatives?
Lecithin, jojoba oil, carnauba wax and rice bran.

FRAGRANCES
Synthetic fragrances are mainly derived from petroleum sources. The word 'fragrance' or 'parfum' on a label can refer to any mixture of synthetic fragrances which may cause allergies, dermatitis and breathing problems.

Look out for (and avoid):
Amyl acetate (banana fragrance), anisole, benzophenones 1 to 12 (rose fragrance), berry fragrance, bitter almond oil (benzaldehyde), cinnamic acid, coconut fragrance, cucumber fragrance, honeysuckle fragrance, lilac fragrance (anisyl acetate), mango fragrance, melon fragrance, methyl acetate (apple fragrance), methyl salicylate (wintergreen or birch fragrance), plum fragrance, peach fragrance, phenethyl alcohol / phenoxyethanol (rose fragrance), strawberry fragrance, vanillin, verataldehyde (vanilla fragrance).

Natural alternatives?
Don't be fooled by 'natural fragrance' – the only way to avoid synthetic fragrances is to stick with certified organic essential oils. Happily, there are masses to choose from.

PRESERVATIVES
Even though nature provides its own preservatives, cosmetics companies favour cheaply produced synthetic equivalents, including parabens, which disrupt hormone levels; and diazolidinyl/imidazoidinyl urea and DMDM hydantoin, which release formaldehyde, a toxic chemical.

Look out for (and avoid):
Ascorbic acid, ascorbyl palmitate, benzethonium chloride, benzyl alcohol, BHA, BHT, boric acid, butyl paraben, captan, cetrimonium bromide, chloramine, chlorhexidine, chlorobutanol, chloroxylenol, chlorphenesin, diazolidinyl urea, DMDM hydantoin, ethanolamines, ethyl paraben, euxyl, germaben, germall, hexachlorophene, imidazolidinyl urea, isopropyl alcohol, kathon, methenamine, methyl paraben, methylisothiazolinone, phenethyl alcohol, phenoxyethanol, phenylphenol, potassium metabisulfite, propyl paraben, quaternary ammonium compounds, salicylic acid, SD alcohol, sodium bisulfite, sodium borate,

sodium hydroxymethylglycinate, sodium propionate, sorbic acid, succinic acid, thimerosal, undecylenic acid.

Natural alternatives?
Tea tree essential oil, thyme essential oil, grapefruit seed extract, bitter orange extract, honey.

SOLVENTS

Water is the most natural solvent (used to dissolve ingredients and extract fragrance) in the world. But not all ingredients dissolve in water, so cosmetics companies may use synthetic solvents instead. These can leave a chemical residue that can irritate the skin, eyes and lungs.

Look out for (and avoid):
Acetic acid, acetone, amyl alcohol, benzene, butylene glycol, ethyl alcohol (synthetic), ethyl butyl acetate, ethylene glycol monophenyl-ether (phenoxyethanol), glycerine, hexane, isopropyl alcohol, methanol, phenol, propyl alcohol, propylene glycol, SD alcohols.

Natural alternatives?
Water, apple cider vinegar, grain alcohol.

SURFACTANTS

Surfactants (surface-acting agents) thicken and create foam in shampoos and skin cleansers. Sodium lauryl sulphate is the poster (bad) boy here and along with DEA, TEA or MEA compounds can irritate the skin and scalp.

Look out for (and avoid):
Ammonium lauryl sulphate, betaine, carboxylate, cocamide DEA or MEA, cocamidopropyl betaine, cocamidopropyl hydroxysultaine, cocamine, cocoamphoglycinate, cococarboxamide MEA-4-carboxylate, coconut and corn oil 'soap', coconut betaine, coconut surfactants (ammonium lauryl or laureth sulphate), coco polyglucose, DEA cetyl phosphate, decyl glucoside, decyl oleate, decyl polyglucose, diethanolamine (DEA), disodium lauryl sulfosuccinate, glyceryl cocoate, glycerol laurate, glycerol monolaurate, glycerol stearate, lactamide DEA, lauramide DEA/MEA, magnesium lauryl sulphate, methyl glucose dioleate, neutralized coconut extract, olefin sulfonate, PEG-100 (polyethylene glycol) stearate, PEG-150 (polyethylene glycol) distearate, sodium coco sulphate, sodium cocoyl isethionate, sodium laureth sulphate, sodium lauryl sulphate, sodium myreth sulphate, sodium myristoyl sarcosinate, sodium stearate, sorbitan stearate, sucrose cocoate, sulphated/sulfonated oil, sodium cocoamphodiacetate, sodium cocoyl glutamate, sodium lauryl sarcosinate, TEA (triethanolamine) lauryl sulphate.

Natural alternatives?
Castile soap (from vegetable oils) and natural foaming agents (yucca extract, soapwort and quillaja bark extract).

THICKENERS

We've been brainwashed to think that thicker creams, shampoos and conditioners are more luxurious but some of the thickening agents carry contamination concerns.

Look out for (and avoid):
Carbomer, cocamide DEA or MEA, hydrolyzed wheat protein, hydroxymethyl cellulose, hydroxypropyl cellulose, methacryloyl ethyl betaine, methacrylates copolymer, oat protein, potassium stearate, quinoa protein, soy protein, vegetable cellulose.

Natural alternatives?
Locust bean gum, guar gum, acacia gum, clay minerals.

Holistically Healthy

As much as I'd like to, I can't blame the cosmetics industry for all my health issues, past, present or future; although it certainly hasn't helped.

Health to me is about balance in all areas – emotional, spiritual, physical, relationships, sexual, intellectual and lifestyle. A former therapist once told me that your life is like an old-fashioned weight scale; for it to function at its best, everything needs to be as closely balanced as possible.

In my quest for perfection, I've read, studied and possibly tried every diet on the face of the Earth; I've been to spiritual classes, Buddhist retreats and Catholic services; tried CBT, ECT and mindful therapy techniques; thrown myself into happy relationships and perhaps even harder into abusive ones; read the dictionary and encyclopaedias and spent hours on Google searching for intellectual stimulus. All of these things aren't bad (except dieting, which I'm not an advocate for) and a lot of them can and do help depending on your situation – but it's been my experience that one without the others is a little like baking a cake without an oven.

I've been fortunate on my journey so far to have had some incredible teachers in various guises, who were either kind and compassionate or cruel and unforgiving; but each one taught me that it's necessary to balance and listen. You are the owner of your body and you are the authority on all things YOU; no one else. Your health is about your balance, and balance (like beauty) is extremely subjective.

Sometimes when I'm not feeling my best I get out my trusty notepad and make a list of everything in my life that makes me happy, even the simple things like being able to brush my teeth or breathe every day, and then I make a second list of things that cause me pain. I'm often surprised that the happy list is always longer than the not-happy one – it's easy to feel like the ceiling is caving in when it's only a little paint that's chipping.

I find that keeping the things that I put into and onto my body as free from worrying chemicals and as close to nature as possible has benefits not just for my body but for my mind. The journey to balance is one only you can take, so I hope some of my advice helps you find your way.

Every Woman's Armour

My friend Veronica (Ronnie) is a makeup artist, and on a few lucky shoots I've had the pleasure of seeing her in action. Everything I've learnt about makeup I've learnt on the job; and if I ever need advice, she's my go-to – just call her Yoda.

Audrey Hepburn once said she liked 'a good hour to dress for a party. I bathe in lavender salts and do my face and then I forget what I look like until the party is over.' My Nan was a bit like that and when I was little I loved to watch her painting her face in the mornings; in fact, her dressing table is still one of the most impressive arrays I've ever seen. Dozens of little glass, apothecary-style jars with creams and powders and colours all laid out in an order I didn't understand; brushes of different sizes and shapes and a beautiful encrusted mirror with fairy-style lights to assist the process. Now my Nan, like all the women in my family, was extraordinarily beautiful with alabaster skin, kind, almond-shaped eyes and a smile that took up her whole face. Even though she didn't need it, every morning the same ritual took place.

One of my first jobs was a before-and-after commercial for a makeup brand, which, incidentally, was where I met Ronnie. First, I posed for the camera *au naturel*, then spent an hour in the chair achieving the so-called 'makeup free' look before posing again with a gleaming smile. I was so excited to see the results of my first real job until I actually saw them – oh my stars! The 'before' shot was horrible – hmm horrible? Let's try DISGUSTING! I'd never really considered myself the most beautiful of creatures but surely I didn't look like that every day?

Thank heavens for good old Ronnie who, while I wept, taught me that 'before' photos are always hideous and there's a reason the red carpet is notorious for layers of carefully constructed makeup.

This book is split the way Ronnie would do it – the skincare (cleanse, tone, moisturize and blemish-bust), then the base, the eyes, the lips and the extras; all the facets to cosmetic perfection. Even now I detest wearing makeup but I know its value, and no matter how comfortable you are in your own skin, sometimes a little armour goes a long way.

X

Easy as One, Two, Three

The recipes are labelled 'easy', 'medium' or 'advanced', so you can see at a glance the amount of time and effort involved. Happily, most of the recipes are a piece of cake – much less work than baking a cake, in fact! Always read through the recipe before you start and be sure you have all the necessary ingredients and equipment to hand.

= Easy
A doddle – you can whip this up in minutes with a few simple ingredients.

= Medium
A little more time and effort required – and maybe the odd specialized ingredient.

= Advanced
Something of a labour of love – but the results are totally worth it!

Every Beauty Cook's Arsenal

If you're going to cook, you're going to need ingredients. These beauty heroes are your staples; you can use them alone, as well as in multiple recipes in this book, and they're easy to find.

Coconut Oil

This wonder ingredient is naturally antibacterial and antifungal, and what's more, it's a brilliant moisturizer, so it's no surprise that it's used as the base of all sorts of natural cosmetics products. Coconut oil is a healthy oil for cooking with, too, and most supermarkets now stock it. I recommend keeping two jars – one in the kitchen and one in the bathroom!

Cocoa Butter

This creamy coloured fat is extracted from the cocoa bean in the process of making chocolate. It's edible, melts at body temperature and its moisturizing powers make it a great addition to natural cosmetics recipes. There's a surprising number of supermarkets that carry cocoa butter as it's quite delicious in cakes and homemade chocolate, but if you can't find it, try a health-food store or online.

Mica Powders

Who would have thought that nature could produce such a dazzling array of colours? Mica powders are derived from the mineral rock muscovite. Once mined, the rock is ground to a fine powder suitable for cosmetic use. Mica powders occur naturally in greys, browns, blues, violets and reds, and may be mixed with iron oxides to produce myriad other colours, too. They are brilliant for adding colour and shimmer to eye shadows and blushers.

Essential Oils

These naturally derived aromatic oils last for years and can be used individually or in a blend to infuse DIY beauty recipes with beautiful fragrance. I purchase them online because it's easier to find all the aromas I want without ever leaving my house. Use those that are certified organic.

Arrowroot Powder

A white starchy powder, made from the rhizomes of the arrowroot plant, *Maranta arundinacea*. Handy to have in the kitchen cupboard for gluten-free baking, it's also a key ingredient in natural deodorant, face powder, and dry shampoo. The cheapest and easiest way to source arrowroot powder is from your local supermarket (if you can't find it, use cornflour instead).

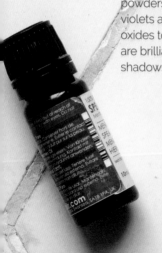

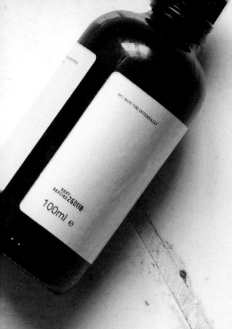

Beeswax

A wondrous natural, non-toxic ingredient which has incredibly useful properties for skincare. It helps to thicken creams and works as a protectant and humectant, providing products with great staying power. I use beeswax in lotions, lotion bars, baby care recipes, lip balm and foot cream. The good stuff has a mild honey scent. Some supermarkets (and even hardware stores) stock this as it's great for polishing wood, but if not, try a health-food store or online.

Liquid Castile Soap

Aside from being a base for heaps of recipes, liquid Castile soap (made from vegetable oils) can actually be used alone for everything. You can clean the house with it, use it as a body or face wash, shampoo, for making baby wipes and much more. Find it online or in health-food stores.

Liquid Carrier Oil

Sometimes you need a thinner base than coconut oil or cocoa butter, and that's where liquid carrier oils come in. I use them for recipes like smoother lotions, baby oil, salves and after-shave balms. My favourites are sweet almond oil and jojoba oil, but you can actually use store-bought extra virgin olive oil.

Shea Butter

This has amazing healing properties and can be used to cure skin rashes and acne; reduce scars, stretch marks, and peeling after tanning; soothe frost bite and burns; and reduce arthritic pain and muscle fatigue. You can find shea butter in health-food stores or online – just make sure it's unscented and unrefined.

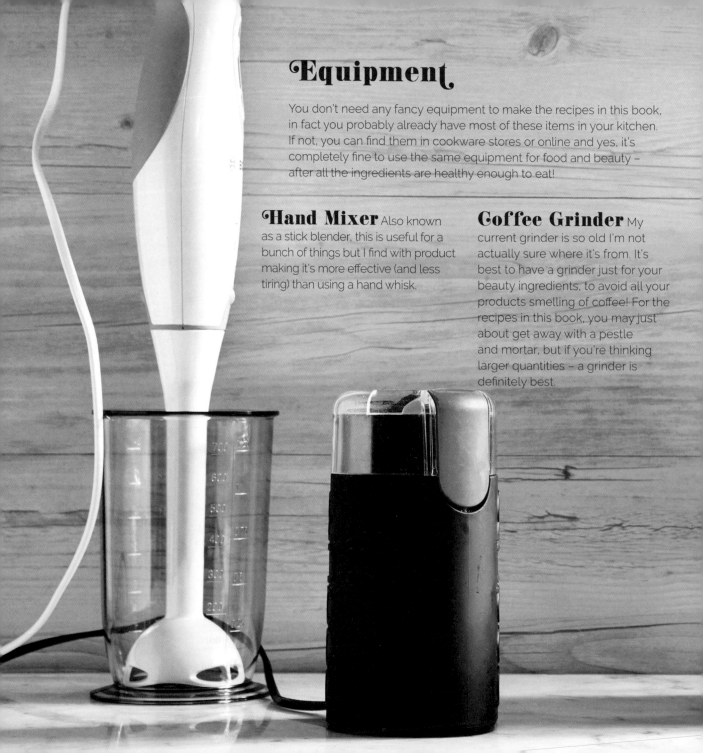

Equipment

You don't need any fancy equipment to make the recipes in this book, in fact you probably already have most of these items in your kitchen. If not, you can find them in cookware stores or online and yes, it's completely fine to use the same equipment for food and beauty – after all the ingredients are healthy enough to eat!

Hand Mixer Also known as a stick blender, this is useful for a bunch of things but I find with product making it's more effective (and less tiring) than using a hand whisk.

Coffee Grinder My current grinder is so old I'm not actually sure where it's from. It's best to have a grinder just for your beauty ingredients, to avoid all your products smelling of coffee! For the recipes in this book, you may just about get away with a pestle and mortar, but if you're thinking larger quantities – a grinder is definitely best.

Water Filter This is really a judgement call. It's not essential, but I prefer to either filter or to once-boil and cool my tap water to remove chlorine and fluoride, which can wreak havoc with your skin, before using the water in my homemade products. If you don't have a filter (or just can't be bothered) using straight tap water is fine.

Measuring Spoons You can pick these up quite easily at any homeware store and my favourites are the set of five sizes all joined together. I recommend using wood or plastic as opposed to metal so there's no need for double sets when it comes to bentonite clay – which can't touch metal EVER! (See safety note, page 28.)

Double Boiler The best way to heat ingredients gently. You simmer water in the lower pan and place the ingredient you want to melt in the upper one. If you don't have a dedicated double boiler, simply place a heatproof bowl over a saucepan and you're good to go. You can allow the water to lap at the bowl, but don't let it flow over the edges of the pan.

Kitchen Scale These are the easiest way to be accurate in your measuring – and digital is best, especially when working with small quantities. Weights don't always have to be exact, but when making some lotions the difference of a gram can change the entire outcome of the recipe.

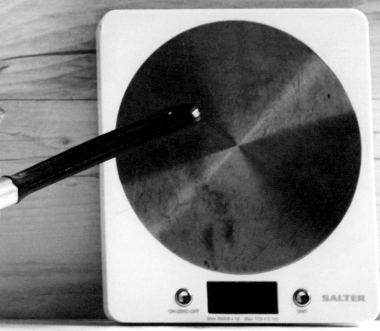

Jars & Bottles & Gifts... Oh My!

It's not necessary to buy specialist tubes or cosmetic containers for your products: any airtight bottles or jars from the pound or dollar store are perfectly fine – even old water bottles will work for your liquid creations. But if you'd like to package your products as gifts or make something that will take pride of place in your bathroom, here are some ideas.

Glass Jars

There's no better way to show off your handiwork than glass jars (plus they're environmentally friendly). Most pound or dollar stores have a variety of these in all shapes, sizes and colours at heavily discounted prices, otherwise homeware stores and some supermarkets stock them, too. When my product is on display it helps for the inside to look as pretty as the outside, so for moisturizers and yummy-looking recipes, I choose clear glass; otherwise opaque or coloured works well. Tie a ribbon around the top, add a handwritten label and you're all set.

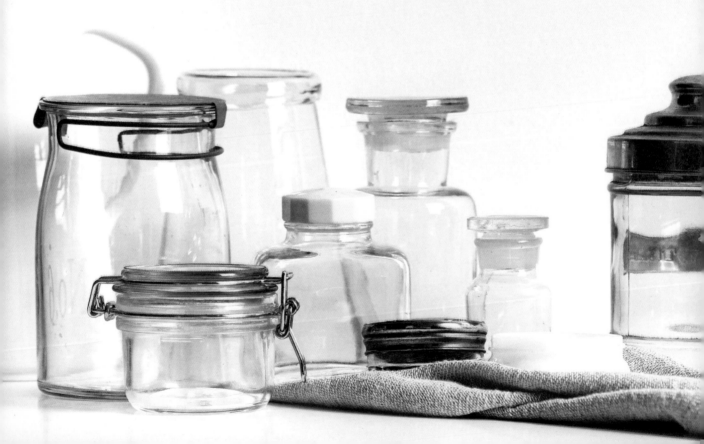

Vases, Pots & Organizers

'Beauty in a pot' is one of the coolest concepts I've ever come across, and while I'd like to take credit for this original idea, it actually belongs to a friend's mum. All over her house she has decorated plant pots holding herbs, spices and powders; vases full of bath salts and bath milk; and organizer pots with chalk-style writing that seem to hold everything else. It's such a clever idea, and as the premise of these recipes is 'all natural', why not use something that signifies nature?

Tubes & Cosmetic Containers

Sometimes a jar is impractical and having my own product line, I know that some things really should be in proper containers. You can buy tubes for homemade lotions and creams online and in some chemists and department stores (just ask for travel cosmetic containers). You can make your own sticky labels and the tubes will fit perfectly in little bags as a set.

Bottles

Reusable spray bottles, pump-top bottles and squeeze bottles are very handy. Glass bottles always look pretty and dark glass bottles are useful to protect essential oils from UV light. Dropper bottles are also brilliant for products that need to be dispensed in small quantities. If you have a home that is top-to-toe tiled, though, just be mindful that if you drop your precious bottle of moisturizer, a glass bottle is more likely to break.

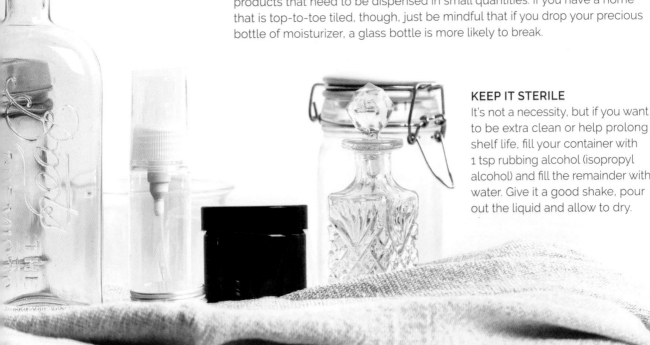

KEEP IT STERILE

It's not a necessity, but if you want to be extra clean or help prolong shelf life, fill your container with 1 tsp rubbing alcohol (isopropyl alcohol) and fill the remainder with water. Give it a good shake, pour out the liquid and allow to dry.

DIY Kilner Jar Foaming Dispenser

1-litre/32fl oz Kilner (Mason) jar
    with screw-top lid
Hammer and nail
Foaming soap dispenser pump
    (I used one from an old soap
    bottle)
Scissors
Couple of rubber bands

I originally made this for the hand wash that sits in my bathroom and next to the kitchen sink, but now I use it for cleansers, moisturizers, shampoo and conditioner and even my body lotion. Kilner (Mason) jars are pretty cheap and you can now find them in several different colours. I usually make my own little labels and cards for these so I remember what's in each one and when I'm using as a gift I customize them with photos and decorations individual to the giftee.

Using a permanent marker, make a mark in the centre of the jar lid. Place the tip of the nail on the mark and use the hammer to tap the nail and pierce a hole. NOTE: the nail can easily slip so please take care!

Use the hammer and nail to make more holes around the first hole, enlarging it until the dispenser pump sits snugly inside.

If the tube of the dispenser is too long for the jar, just trim it with a pair of scissors so it doesn't quite reach the bottom of the jar.

Wind a rubber band around the pump dispenser, directly under the lid. This is to form a seal to stop any soap escaping in case the jar tips over. You may need to add another rubber band to make a good seal.

Fill the jar with your product and screw on the lid.

#everyonelovesaquickie These days lots of stationery and discount stores sell glass 'drinking' jars with a hole pre-made for a straw. In the world of homemade beauty, these remove the need for hammer and nail, providing the perfect pre-perforated lid for a pump dispenser. Use an elastic band to create a seal around the pump stem if you need to.

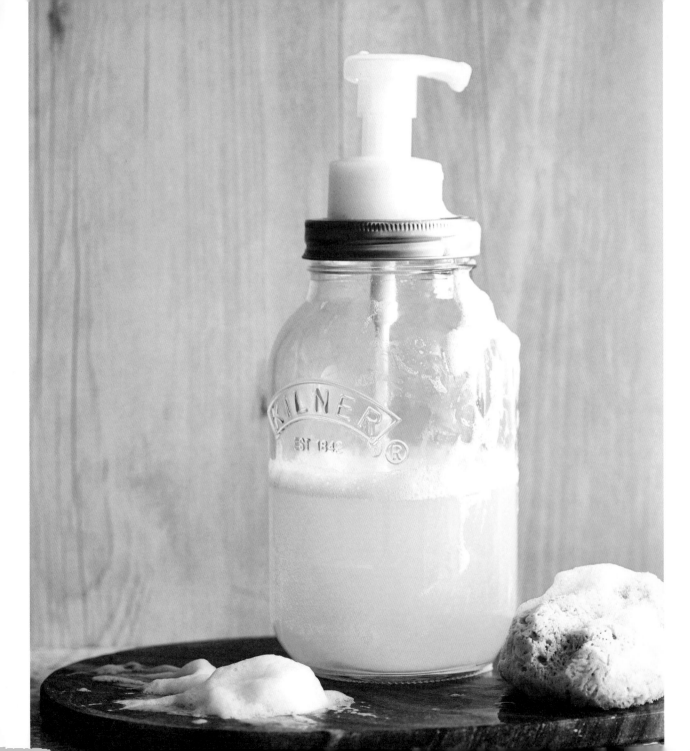

What is my Skin Type?

Just as no two people have exactly the same eye colour, none of us has exactly the same skin type as the next person. But, if you had to put a label on it, we do all have skin that falls into broad categories, and this is how the beauty industry helps us to choose the 'right' products. The following three-step process will help you to get to grips with your own skin type right now – but remember, it could change as you age, and even with the seasons and the weather! Retest every now and then to make sure what you're using is still what your skin needs.

STEP 1

Cleanse your skin using one of the gentle #quickies on pages 32–3. Then, rinse with fresh water and use a clean facecloth to pat dry. Now, without touching your face at all (sit on your hands or take up knitting if you have to), wait for your skin to settle down into its own 'normal' – an hour should do it.

STEP 2

Take a clean, white tissue (not the kind with balm on – just a plain one) and fold it into a square to fit your face. Hold the edges and pat it down across your forehead, and round your eyes and your nose. Then, across your chin. Set aside the tissue, but don't throw it away. Find a hand-held mirror (one of those magnifying ones is perfect). Then use Step 3 to make your skin-type assessment.

STEP 3

Which of the following best describes what you see on your tissue and in the mirror?

No flakes of skin or oily residue appear on the tissue. The skin on your face looks clear. You have:
Normal Skin

Small grease spots appear on the tissue; in the mirror you can see open pores and your skin has an oily sheen. You have:
Oily Skin

You can see flakes of skin on your face or on the tissue and your face looks tight, with tiny pores. It probably feels tight, too. You have:
Dry Skin

There are mixed signals on the tissue – some grease spots, some flakes; in the mirror, you have areas of open pores and of tightness. You have:
Combination Skin

Three Steps to Beautiful Skin

There are only two places on your body where your skin doesn't produce sebum (the body's natural lubricant): the palms of your hands and the soles of your feet. Other than that, your skin is an oil-making machine of immense proportions. Most people have a love/hate relationship with sebum; too much and you're probably the shiny, pimply kid in the corner of the playground (hello seventh grade), but too little and your skin will be flaky, cracked and old before its time.

As well as providing lubrication, sebum contributes to the barrier that protects your skin from pollutants. And your body knows its value, so strip off sebum with harsh products and up goes production (again, it's a love/hate thing).

The skin itself is a complex, multi-layered organ – the largest organ in the body, in fact. Sometimes, you need to nurture it and really care for it so that it can look its best. This three-step system works on the three areas that influence your journey to beautiful, healthy skin – pollutants, pH and moisture.

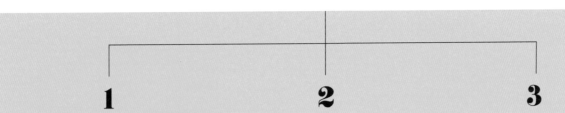

1

CLEANSE (aka to clean)
The purpose of a cleanser is to remove impurities. When the body is stressed (from mental stress, exercise or anything that raises the heart rate), it produces extra sebum. Couple this with pollutants in the atmosphere – car fumes, cigarette smoke and a generous layer of makeup – and you've got skin that's dirty. This dirt clogs the pores and stops the natural cell turnover that is important for youthful and healthy skin. A cleanser detoxifies this topical nightmare.

2

TONE (aka to restore)
The original purpose of toning was to restore the skin's natural pH (that is, its relative acid–alkaline balance), which should sit around the 5–7 mark (slightly alkaline – the same number recommended for your whole body). Toning also tightens and shrinks enlarged pores, returning them to more normal proportions; ensures any leftover toxic debris is removed; and helps get rid of the dead cells and dirt that cause acne.

3

MOISTURIZE (aka to nourish)
A moisturizer has two roles. First, it nourishes your skin. That is, you can expect it to soothe, hydrate and replenish lost moisture. Second, it protects your skin against external irritants: basically, it acts as a barrier to keep out toxins, pollutants and any other nasties in the air.

Glossary

Alcohol Manufactured by fermenting sugars, widely used in perfumes, bathroom products and cosmetics and for making herbal medicines.

Allantoin A naturally occurring compound found in the comfrey plant. It helps heal wounds and skin ulcers.

Aloe Vera One of the most multi-tasking, health-promoting plants on Earth and can be both ingested and applied topically. It comes in juice, gel and powder forms.

Amino Acids There are 22 known amino acids, eight of which can't be produced by the body, and these are called essential amino acids. The body needs them in order to create its own proteins. In beauty products, amino acids are used to aid the metabolic processes in the skin and hair to repair and improve their condition.

Antioxidants Food compounds that neutralize chemicals called free radicals.

Apple Cider Vinegar The only alkaline vinegar, made by fermenting apple cider.

Arrowroot Powder A white, powdery starch that comes from tropical plants: the most common being *Maranta arundinacea*.

Bee Pollen This granular garnish is made by worker bees, who pack pollen into little granules with added honey or nectar.

Bicarbonate of Soda (Baking Soda) Bicarbonate of soda is a component of a natural mineral called natron which is found in mineral springs. It can be used for just about anything from deodorizing your shoes to easing indigestion.

Clays Fine-grained natural rock or soil material. Clay comes in different colours and varieties, including bentonite, kaolin and Australian beige clay.

Bentonite Clay
A WARNING!
Bentonite clay is a positively charged element, which means it attaches to negative elements. If it comes into contact with anything metallic, it becomes toxic. Use glass bowls and wooden or plastic utensils for all recipes containing bentonite.

Cocoa Butter An edible, ultra-hydrating vegetable fat that is derived from the cocoa bean, which also gives us chocolate.

Emulsifying Wax (Vegetable Derived) A non-toxic emulsifier used in cosmetics to produce lotions and creams.

Essential Fatty Acid An essential fat that the body can't manufacture itself. EFA deficiency can lead to kidney and liver damage, anaemia, eczema, inflammations of the skin and hair, scaling and more.

Essential Oil This is a concentrated liquid containing aroma compounds from plants. Essential oils are used mostly as a fragrance, but also have benefits individual to the plant used.

Grapeseed Oil Extracted from the seeds of grapes, grapeseed oil has strong antibacterial and antioxidant properties.

Honey (Raw) Derived from sustainable producers it maintains the moisture level in the skin and has antiseptic and antibacterial properties. Best to use raw if you can find it so you're getting straight honey with no alterations or additions.

Jojoba Oil Extracted from the seeds of the jojoba plant, this waxy oil is similar in nature to our own sebum. It helps to lubricate and protect the skin.

Keratin A protein found in our hair, nails and skin and in the horns, hooves and claws of other mammals. Most commonly added to hair products to give strength and smoothness.

Macrobiotic Sea Salt This is made by the action of sun and wind on sea water.

Magnesium A naturally occurring salt used as a thickener, colouring or anticaking agent. Magnesium sulphate is often known as Epsom salts and is used to ease muscle tension and stress and to reduce certain seizures.

Peptides Shorter chains of amino acids combined to create proteins, these target wrinkles and aging of the skin.

Saponification The process of making a fatty acid into a salt by treating with an alkali; to saponify is to convert to soap.

Saponin A natural glycoside (sugar compound) that occurs in plants, such as sarsaparilla. It is mainly used as a foaming agent.

Shea Butter Derived from the fruit of the karate tree, shea butter is deeply moisturizing, softening and nourishing and leaves a protective film on the skin.

Tea Tree Oil A steam distilled from the leaves and flowers of the tea tree, this has strong antibacterial and antiseptic properties.

Vegetable Glycerine A thick, syrupy substance present in the fats and oils of vegetables. It helps to hydrate, soften and soothe the skin and assist in the retention of moisture.

Waxes (Beeswax, Soy Wax, Calendilla Wax) Obtained from animals, insects and plants though there are also mineral and synthetic waxes. Chemically, they are mostly a compound of various fatty acids, and are less greasy than fats or butters. To remove household spills requires a solvent – the best is turpentine as it dissolves wax completely.

Zinc A chemical element (Zn), mostly used as a protective coating to other metals. Zinc is an essential element in the growth of many organisms, both plant and animal. A deficiency in zinc in humans has been found to stunt growth and contribute to anaemia.

Zinc Oxide A naturally occurring mineral, used as an antiseptic, astringent and in protective creams like sunblock.

CLEANSERS

#keepitclean

One of my favourite things at the end of the day is washing my face.
All the stress goes down the drain with the water and it's a great way to
be in the moment and do something that's just for me.

I think I was about 12 when I first started using a cleanser every day and I've spent
years finding the perfect one – strong enough to clean deeply, but still gentle on
the skin. Unfortunately, I wasn't gifted with my mothers' naturally blemish-free skin
and had more pimples growing up than I could count on both my hands. Before I
began making my own products, I probably tested all (or at least close to all) the
products on the market, so I know the feeling of dissatisfaction when something
doesn't work. I don't want a solution that causes a hundred other problems; frankly,
I don't have the time. In my job, getting hired (or fired) can come down to the
quality of your skin. Even if your work isn't quite so cut-throat, I know you want the
same as I do – one answer, one solution, one complete cure-all!

The recipes in this chapter are exactly that (no fine print required).

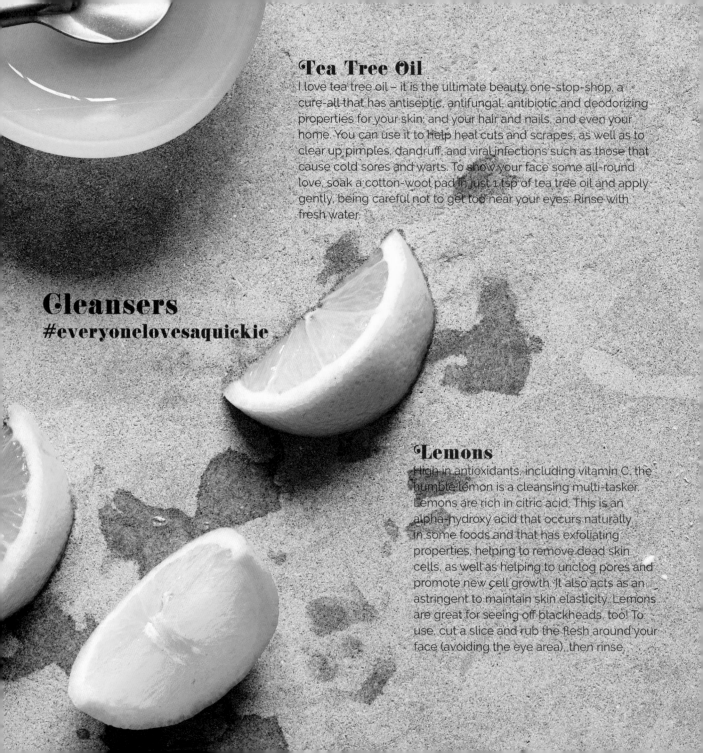

Tea Tree Oil

I love tea tree oil – it is the ultimate beauty one-stop-shop, a cure-all that has antiseptic, antifungal, antibiotic and deodorizing properties for your skin, and your hair and nails, and even your home. You can use it to help heal cuts and scrapes, as well as to clear up pimples, dandruff, and viral infections such as those that cause cold sores and warts. To show your face some all-round love, soak a cotton-wool pad in just 1 tsp of tea tree oil and apply gently, being careful not to get too near your eyes. Rinse with fresh water.

Cleansers
#everyonelovesaquickie

Lemons

High in antioxidants, including vitamin C, the humble lemon is a cleansing multi-tasker. Lemons are rich in citric acid. This is an alpha-hydroxy acid that occurs naturally in some foods and that has exfoliating properties, helping to remove dead skin cells, as well as helping to unclog pores and promote new cell growth. It also acts as an astringent to maintain skin elasticity. Lemons are great for seeing off blackheads, too! To use, cut a slice and rub the flesh around your face (avoiding the eye area), then rinse.

Yogurt

The ultimate DIY face mask, natural yogurt (avoid the fruit-flavoured versions) is rich in lactic acid, which is an emollient, meaning it helps to smooth out the skin; and healthy bacteria, which help to repair the damage caused by environmental toxins and even sunlight. Finally, lactic acid, just like citric (see opposite, below), is an alpha-hydroxy acid, which helps to exfoliate the skin, minimize blemishes, and reduce the signs of aging. To use, massage a dollop of yogurt into your skin (avoiding the eye area), then rinse.

Bicarbonate of Soda (Baking Soda)

This is probably the most underrated ingredient you already have in your pantry. It costs less than a buck (quid/euro/you get the gist), you can use it all around your house (not just on your skin), it's edible so there's no stress if you accidentally swallow some and it's environmentally friendly. As a cleanser it's unparalleled, it doesn't dehydrate the skin or strip away healthy oils but removes dead cells and unclogs pores. It's also a natural deodorizer so no icky smells. To use, dilute 1 tsp of bicarbonate of soda in 1 tbsp warm water, then gently massage the mixture into your skin (avoiding the eye area) and rinse.

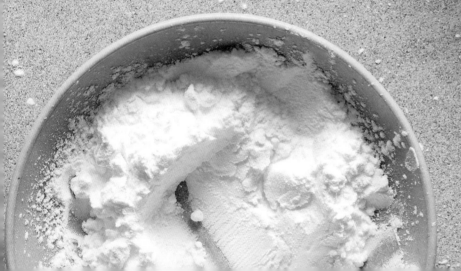

Gentle Agave Face Wash

This is my go-to cleanser and it was one of the first recipes I ever made. The ingredients are both nourishing and hardworking, everything a great cleanser should be. Suitable for all skin types, it is antiseptic, antifungal, healing and soothing, making it nigh-on perfect. This version is also vegan. **Bonus** – it takes less than 5 minutes to make.

Makes about 375ml/13fl oz/ 1½ cups
Shelf life: 6 months

60ml/2fl oz/¼ cup liquid Castile soap
5 tsp sweet almond oil
2 tbsp agave
15 drops elemi essential oil
15 drops lemon essential oil

Measure 250ml/9fl oz/1 cup of filtered water into a jug, then add the liquid Castile soap, followed by the sweet almond oil, agave and the essential oils. Gently stir everything together until the mixture is fully combined and it has turned cloudy. Pour the mixture into a foaming dispenser (such as the DIY Kilner jar on page 24).

To use, shake well, then dispense a few pumps into the palm of your hand, rub your hands together to create a foam and massage gently over your face and neck. Rinse well with warm water.

WEEKLY CLEAN AND POLISH

EVERYDAY OILING

We go to such pains to avoid having 'oily skin' that it can seem counterintuitive to actually choose to put oil on the face. However, improving the quality of your skin sometimes needs just that to get those sebaceous glands working properly. Castor oil and extra-virgin olive oil are all you need. Use equal parts if you have normal or combination skin; up the castor oil a little if you have oily skin (castor oil can help to unclog the pores of backed-up sebum and debris); and up the olive oil, with its fabulous moisturizing properties, if you have dry or chapped skin.

HOW TO USE: Mix small amounts of the castor and olive oils in your chosen proportions in a bowl. When I say small amounts, I mean tiny – a little goes a long way (think in half-teaspoons). Wash your face and pat it dry with a clean facecloth. Then dip your fingertips in the oil mixture and apply to your skin – smoothing it out over your face and rubbing it in evenly. Take your clean facecloth and run it under warm water, wring it out so that it's just damp and lay it over your face. Relax. Stay like that for 5–10 minutes, then remove the facecloth and rinse your face in fresh water and pat dry. Do this every day and within a week, your skin should start to appear healthier, and your pores should be clear.

WEEKLY FRIDGE RETREAT

Okay, I confess: this isn't about diving into the fridge and finding that chocolate pudding you've been saving for a rainy day. No, instead, every week raid your fridge and save your skin: with just an avocado and a lemon and a couple of slices of cucumber – no need for anything more.

HOW TO USE: Mash up the avocado flesh with 2 tbsp of juice from the lemon. Wash and cleanse your face, and pat dry with a clean facecloth or towel. Then, use your clean hands to smear the avocado and lemon mixture all over your face, avoiding your eyes (it won't damage them, but it will sting – just rinse it out with fresh water if your eyes inadvertently get hit). Now, because I want you to relax (this is a retreat, remember), use a natural eye mask – two slices of cucumber, one over each eye (cucumber has properties that help to sooth inflammation, so can help to reduce puffiness in the lids and around your eyes). Lie back and allow the avocado and lemon face mask to dry up – at least 20 minutes. When you're ready, remove the cucumber slices, the wash off the face mask with fresh water and pat your skin dry. Glorious!

Coconut & Citrus Cream Cleanser

If you've got dry skin, it's the middle of winter or your face feels a little like an old pair of shoes, then this cleanser is for you. I quite often use this one at night, especially during the colder months when the skin so easily loses moisture and it's even more important to keep it buffed and hydrated. The lemon and witch hazel in this cleanser unclog pores and remove dirt, while the oil and wax nourish and restore moisture.

Makes about 100ml/3½fl oz/
⅓ cup + 2 tbsp
Shelf life: 6 weeks

1 tbsp beeswax
2 tbsp coconut oil
10g/¼oz cocoa butter
1 tbsp lemon juice
1 tbsp witch hazel
1 large pinch of bicarbonate of soda
    (baking soda)
6 drops sweet orange essential oil

Make a double boiler by placing a glass bowl over a pan of simmering water. Allow the water to lap at the bowl, but not to flow over the edges of the pan. Add the beeswax, coconut oil and cocoa butter, allow to melt, then remove the bowl (take care – the bowl will be hot) and set aside to cool slightly, just until it has started to re-solidify and is soft set. Use a hand mixer to beat the wax and oil mixture until it is fully combined and you have a creamy consistency, about 3–5 minutes.

Put the lemon juice and witch hazel in another heatproof bowl and set it over the double boiler – allow it to heat until just warm (it shouldn't take more than 5 minutes, so keep an eye on it because if you heat the mixture too much, the witch hazel will evaporate), then remove the bowl from the pan and stir in the bicarbonate of soda.

Add the lemon and witch hazel mixture to the oil mixture a little at a time, beating with a wooden spoon or spatula between each addition to make sure everything is combined. Allow to cool completely, then add the sweet orange essential oil and beat again. Transfer to an airtight container to store.

To use, apply a thin layer of the cream to your face and neck (rubbing the mixture between your hands to soften it, if necessary), then soak a muslin cloth in hand-hot water and gently wipe your face to remove the cream.

*If you're using coconut oil and want to gift this, you can buy little faux coconuts online. Attach a ribbon and you've got something special.

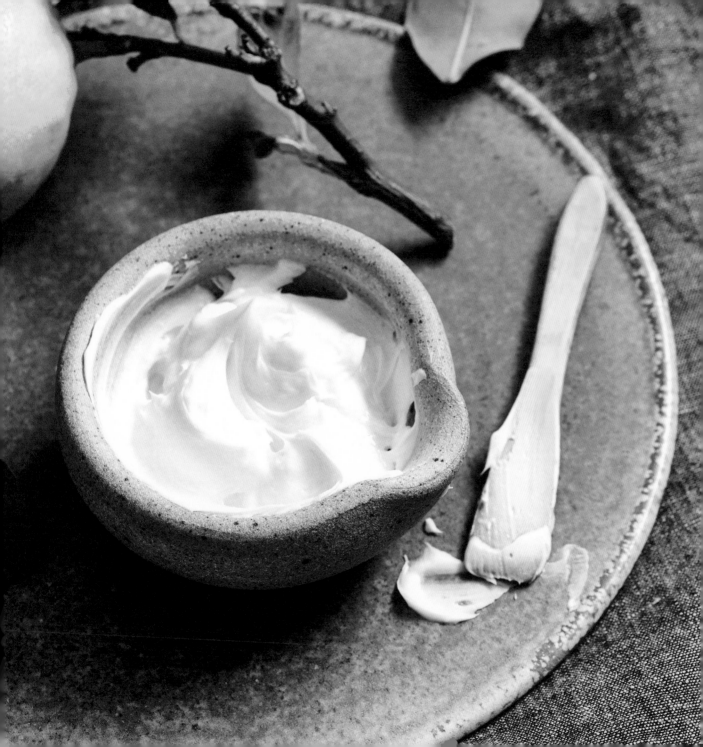

Scented Witch Hazel Makeup Remover

By now I've seen way too many previews of what happens when you leave your makeup on overnight and believe me it's not pretty! Clogged pores and a bland complexion are just the start, and who wants to look old before their time? This recipe is perfect for clearing away your 'work face' and soothing the skin so that it can repair while you sleep.

Makes about 90ml/3fl oz/
⅓ cup + 1 tbsp
Shelf life: 6 months

2 tbsp witch hazel
2 tbsp kukui nut oil
2 drops lavender or rose geranium
    essential oil

Put 2 tbsp of filtered water into a small bottle and add the witch hazel, kukui nut oil and lavender or rose geranium essential oil. Put the lid on the bottle and shake well to fully combine. To use, shake again and then soak a cotton-wool pad or ball in the mixture and gently pass over your skin.

*Kukui nut oil comes from the candlenut tree, which is native to Hawaii. The oil has incredible, restorative properties and has been used for centuries to treat wounds, burns, eczema, psoriasis and scarring. It's also great for soothing sunburn – apply a small amount to the affected area and allow to soak into the skin.

The Oil Cleansing Method

We are constantly being told that washing our hair too often strips it of its natural oils and makes it look dull and lifeless. If that's true for our hair, then the same principle applies to our skin. Water-washing, day in day out, strips the skin of its natural lubricants. This can have one of two effects (and often a combination of both): the skin dries out and looks dull and lifeless (sound familiar?) and/or the sebaceous glands go into overdrive to correct the dryness and produce more oil than the skin needs – that shiny, greasy look. So, how about, rather than turning to water as a cleanser, we look to natural oils that are much closer to the oils the skin itself produces?

Oil Cleansing Combos

There's no one-size-fits all when it comes to oil cleansing, but here are some of my favourite combinations for each skin type. Feel free to experiment until you find what works for you. These oils will keep for a few weeks in a sealed container.

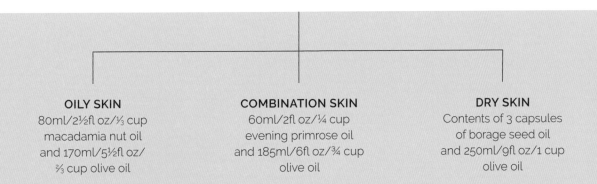

OILY SKIN
80ml/2½fl oz/⅓ cup
macadamia nut oil
and 170ml/5½fl oz/
⅔ cup olive oil

COMBINATION SKIN
60ml/2fl oz/¼ cup
evening primrose oil
and 185ml/6fl oz/¾ cup
olive oil

DRY SKIN
Contents of 3 capsules
of borage seed oil
and 250ml/9fl oz/1 cup
olive oil

HOW TO USE
Rinse your face with fresh water and pat dry with a clean facecloth. Rub a little of your chosen oil mixture between the palms of your hands and massage the oil into your skin, using small circular motions all over your face, and not forgetting across your brow and over your chin. When you're ready, wet the facecloth with warm water and wring it out so that it's damp. Place it over your face and leave it there for a minute or two, then gently pull it away and pat your face dry with a clean towel.

TONERS
#timetorestore

There's no right or wrong when it comes to toner versus mist (spritz) – it's really up to the individual. In my product line, I make mists, but a mist is really just a toner in a spray bottle. If you're travelling or short on time, a quick spritz is easier than finding a cotton-wool pad or a tissue to apply your toner, but if you're using the somewhat old-school application, you're probably far more thorough. The only essential here is that you actually complete this part of your three-step routine.

You can use any of these recipes as a straight toner or a spritz, depending on the bottle you use or if you're packaging them up as gifts.

If you're applying straight to the skin, soak a cotton-wool pad in the liquid and wipe gently over your face. If you're a sprayer, then make sure you spritz your whole face (one spray is not enough – you'll need four or five).

Old-school, new-school or somewhere in between, it's all about you, so take time to restore.

X

Apple Cider Vinegar

Apple cider vinegar (ACV) contains alpha hydroxy acid, a naturally occurring fruit acid that has been used for centuries as an exfoliant – clearing the skin of dead cells and other debris. In addition, ACV balances the natural pH levels of the skin, and helps to even out the appearance of age spots, wrinkles and even sun damage. You can find it in supermarkets, and it's super-cheap, which makes it pretty much perfect as #quickies go. To use, mix 1 part ACV to 2 parts water and use a cotton-wool pad to apply, avoiding your eyes.

Toners
#everyonelovesaquickie

Green Tea

Often touted as a superfood, green tea can also improve your complexion. It reduces excess oil production, calms rosacea and redness, tightens the pores, refines the skin, soothes irritated blemishes, replenishes moisture and gives an all-round glow. There are two ways to use this as a toner:

Option 1 Brew the tea, let it cool, then freeze in ice-cube trays. To use, pop out a cube and use it to 'wipe' your face.

Option 2 Brew the tea, let it cool, then remove the tea bag and use the tea bag to wipe your face.

Witch Hazel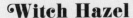

Witch hazel contains tannins (a textural element that causes dryness), so it acts as a natural astringent. For acne-prone skin, it reduces inflammation and excess oil; you can also soak two cotton-wool pads in it, then apply to closed eyes for 5 minutes to reduce puffiness. It can heal bruises, reduce varicose veins, remove impurities, help lock in moisture, treat razor burns, ease eczema and even soothe sunburn. If you're looking for something loaded with skincare benefits that's eco-friendly and cheap, you can't get better than this classic. To use, soak a cotton-wool pad in witch hazel and apply to your skin before moisturizing.

Rose Water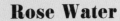

This is by far one of the most amazing ingredients you can add to your beauty regime. It helps maintain the skin's natural pH balance; fights acne, dermatitis and eczema; heals scars, cuts and wounds; helps hydrate and soothe the skin; is antibacterial; relieves stress and anxiety and is high in antioxidants to strengthen skin cells and improve their regeneration. To use, place a few drops on a cotton-wool pad and apply to your skin.

Homemade Rose Water

1 rose makes about 100ml/
3½fl oz/⅓ cup + 2 tbsp
Shelf life: 1 month (see tip below)

Roses (the more you use, the more
water you make, so the choice is
yours based on the shelf life and
your usage)

I like my rose water as fresh as possible, and there's nothing fresher than making your own. This is a simple DIY you can use yourself or give as a gift (the smell is amazing and no one has to know it wasn't hard work). You can use this as a refreshing toner or a hair rinse, or add a few drops to your bath water to help nourish your skin cells.

Store-bought rose water can be extremely overpriced and filled with artificial ingredients, so if you are going to buy it, please make sure it's 100-per-cent pure with no additions.

Pick the petals from the rose stalks and discard the stalks and leaves. Place the petals in a saucepan and cover with filtered water. Use 100ml/3½fl oz water per rose – that is, two roses = 200ml/7fl oz water.

Cover the pan with a lid and place it over a low heat. Bring the water up to a gentle simmer (take care not to let it boil) and then continue to simmer for 30–40 minutes, always checking that things aren't getting too fierce. You will notice the petals losing their colour and an oil residue forming on the surface of the water.

Place a fine kitchen strainer, a muslin or a cheesecloth over a bowl and strain the mixture. Discard the petals and let the water cool completely. Transfer the rose water to a glass jar and store in a cool, dark place. (See page 43 for how to use just as it is.)

*Adding 1 tsp of vitamin E oil to the mixture before storing will extend the shelf life by 2 months (so, it will last for 3 months altogether).

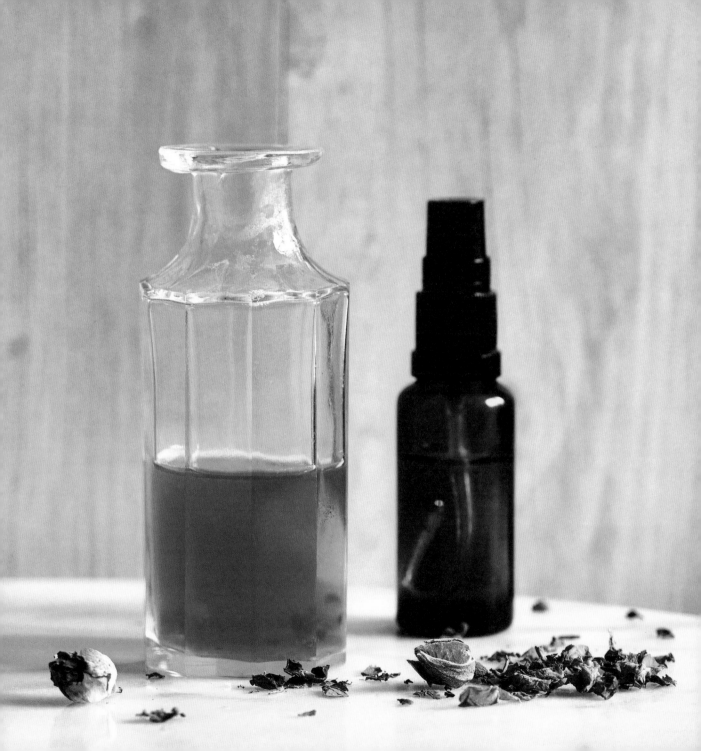

Protective Rose Water Face Mist

Rose water by itself is great for your skin, but with the addition of witch hazel and carrot seed it can do even more. This mist works well for all skin types, hydrating and purifying at the same time, as well as helping to protect against sun damage. I love to use this in the evenings to relax me and really soothe my skin after a long day.

Makes about 250ml/9fl oz/1 cup
Shelf life: 3 months

125ml/4fl oz/½ cup rose water
   (see page 44)
1 tsp witch hazel
5 drops carrot seed essential oil

Using a funnel, pour 125ml/4fl oz/½ cup filtered water into a spray bottle, then add the rose water, witch hazel and carrot seed essential oil. Shake the mixture to combine fully, replace the lid and store in a cool, dark place, such as a bathroom cabinet. To use, shake up the bottle, then simply spritz your face with four or five pumps at the end of your cleansing routine.

Simple Citrus Face Spritz

If I were allowed to use only one mist, it would be this one. A spritz at the start of the day is all I need to get me energized. It is rich in vitamin C, which is essential for the body's production of collagen (the binder that gives the skin its elasticity) and a superhero antioxidant that fights damage from free radicals to rejuvenate aged and tired skin and help maintain a firm and youthful appearance (like I said, it's my favourite).

Makes about 250ml/9fl oz/1 cup
Shelf life: 3 months

1 orange
1 lemon
2 grapefruits
½ tsp vitamin E oil

Using a vegetable peeler, carefully remove the zest of each of the fruit – you want the zest, rather than the pith, so think fine slivers of peel, rather than thick chunks. Place the zest in a heatproof glass measuring jug and pour over 250ml/9fl oz/1 cup of boiling water. Cover the jug with a clean tea towel and leave to steep for 12–24 hours. (Now would be a good time to make yourself a fruit salad with the discarded flesh of the fruit.)

Pour the citrus water through a fine sieve into a clean measuring jug or a bowl with a pouring spout. Discard the zest. Add the vitamin E oil to the citrus water, stir to combine and pour the mixture into a spray bottle. To use, shake up the bottle, then simply spritz your face with four or five pumps at the end of your cleansing routine.

Dandelion Leaf Toner

Who would've thought a humble weed could have magical powers for the skin: dandelion has properties that are wonderful for removing impurities that are the enemy of a clear complexion. Combining the leaf with nourishing, skin-enhancing essential oils and age-busting bee propolis means that this toner is everything a girl (or boy) needs for wholehearted rejuvenation. I love to use this toner during my busy times (mostly Fashion Week), when my skin is being subjected to copious amounts of makeup and to applicators that aren't always properly cleaned. Think of this as an antibiotic for your skin.

Makes about 300ml/10½fl oz/
   1 cup + 3 tbsp
Shelf life: 3 months

125ml/4fl oz/½ cup cooled
   dandelion leaf tea
125ml/4fl oz/½ cup witch hazel
20 drops alcohol-free bee propolis
   tincture
1 tbsp lemon juice
2 tbsp aloe vera juice
1 tbsp jojoba oil
20 drops lavender essential oil
20 drops geranium essential oil
10 drops mandarin essential oil

Pour the tea into a small bowl and add the witch hazel, bee propolis and lemon juice. Stir well to combine. Add the aloe vera juice (this will help the oils mix into the tea without separating), the jojoba oil and the essential oils, then stir well to combine again. Decant the mixture into one or two cosmetics bottles and store in a cool, dark place. To use, shake the bottle, then simply soak a cotton-wool pad or ball in the toner and apply to your skin.

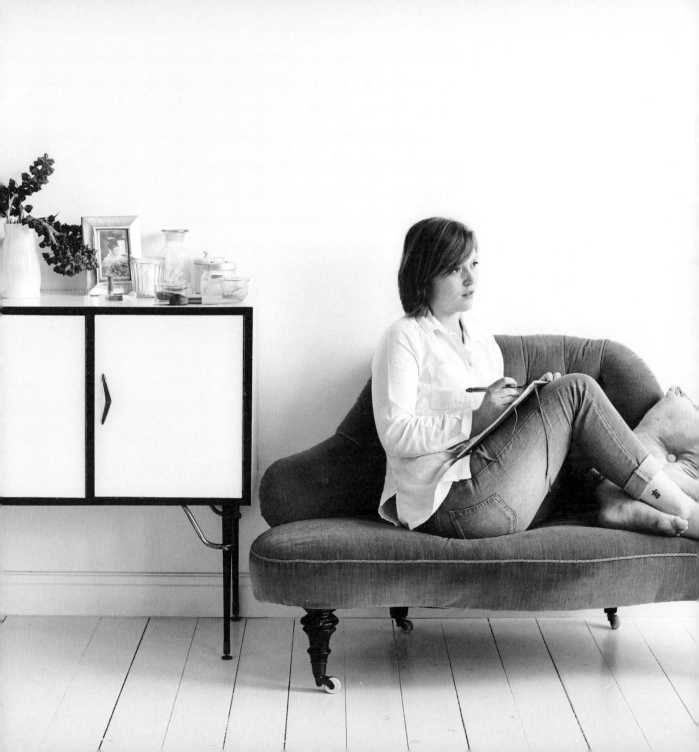

MOISTURIZERS
#nourishnaturally

If you walk down the skincare aisle in any grocery store, you'll see whole shelves devoted to lotions, potions and creams. Some claim to be a miracle cure for wrinkles, while others are designed to be oil-free for teenage skin; some have SPF to protect you during the day, while others are formulated for the evening or night.

In my industry, thousands upon thousands of dollars are spent every year on creating (and marketing) moisturizers for the general public. The question I'm most often asked is: if the price is high, does it mean it's better for you? Short answer – NO!

Price doesn't equate to quality when it comes to moisturizers. Most brands spend around £2.50/$3.50 US/$5 AUS to fill their jars 'en masse', so what you're really paying for (aside from a bunch of dubious chemicals), is the privilege of using a brand-named product.

So, what can you do? Nourishing your skin, while being essential, is also super easy: it's actually the easiest part of the three-step system. Anything with a pure oil count will pretty much do the trick. It's about replacing lost moisture and protecting the outer layers from penetration by pollutants. I promise it's not rocket science (although it feels like it when you're reading the back of those perfect little jars). Any of these recipes will work wonders; and if you're short on time, just use a spoonful of any of the ingredients listed in #everyonelovesaquickie.

X

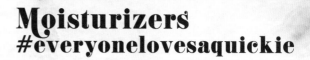

Moisturizers
#everyonelovesaquickie

Coconut Oil

So many natural beauty products use coconut oil, and for good reason: it is naturally antibacterial and antifungal, is an excellent moisturizer, can penetrate better than other oils and, well, smells like cookies. You can use it for soothing dry hands, as a cheekbone highlighter, to shave your legs, as a hair conditioner and even to remove eye makeup. It also stops moisture loss, so is particularly good for older skin that tends to dry out more rapidly. To use, rub ½–1 tsp of raw, unrefined coconut oil in your palm to soften, then apply to your face.

Shea Butter

Brimming with essential fatty acids and plant sterols, shea butter has amazing healing properties. It can heal skin rashes, peeling after tanning, scars, stretch marks, frostbite, acne and burns, and ease the pain of arthritis and muscle fatigue. It's also high in vitamins A and E, which protect the cells from free radicals and environmental damage, and assist the skin in maintaining its elasticity. Plus, shea butter protects against ultraviolet radiation so it acts as a natural sunscreen. To use, place ½–1 tsp of raw, unprocessed shea butter in your palm and apply to your face.

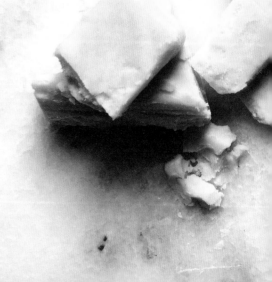

Argan Oil

Imagine fruit so nutritious that goats will climb trees just to eat them! Inside such a fruit is the little nut that gives us argan oil. Originating from Morocco, it's now used all around the world as an effective, all-natural moisturizer for skin and hair, as well as to treat infections, bug bites and skin rashes. Packed full of omega-6 fatty acids and vitamins A and E, it helps boost cell production and fight off aging. As a moisturizer, it's quick to absorb, is non-greasy and reduces fine lines and wrinkles. To use, place a few drops of argan oil in your palm and gently massage into the skin.

Aloe Vera

This all-rounder contains two hormones: auxins and gibberellins. These have wound-healing and anti-inflammatory properties that reduce inflammation. Gibberellin also acts as a growth hormone, stimulating the production of new cells, which allows skin to heal faster. It's soothing, fights aging, reduces the appearance of stretch marks and helps clear up acne-prone skin. To use, take a large dollop of aloe vera gel and apply as you would a moisturizer (to make this extra potent, you can add a few drops of vitamin E oil).

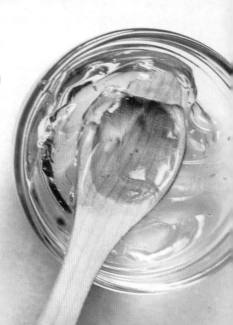

Super-easy Repair & Protect Face Cream

Makes about 125ml/4fl oz/½ cup
Shelf life: 12 months

125ml/4fl oz/½ cup melted
    coconut oil
1 tsp extra-virgin olive oil
5–7 drops rose geranium or
    lavender essential oil

Extra-virgin olive oil contains vitamin E – a powerful antioxidant that neutralizes the effects of skin-damaging free radicals that break down collagen to weaken the skin's elasticity, and cause skin dryness and wrinkles. In short, extra-virgin olive oil repairs and protects the skin. Tick and tick!

  I've given you a choice of two essential oils. Both are soothing, repairing purifying and smell great; in fact the scents alone have been shown to reduce anxiety, irritability and symptoms of depression (#winningformula). You'll find it easier to get hold of lavender than rose geranium, but lavender can react with very sensitive skin. In fact, nothing divides the 'au-naturel' community quite like this little purple flower. Personally, I love it – I've never had an adverse reaction and I usually have extremely sensitive skin, but I do recommend a patch test if you're a newbie to the lavender world. Two drops of essential oil on the inside of your wrist will do – if the oil doesn't agree with you, you will know (don't worry – a dollop of aloe vera gel over the patch will clear up any reaction).

Combine all the ingredients in a bowl. Mix thoroughly and transfer to an airtight container (it couldn't really be any easier). A little goes a long way: to use, rub a small amount of moisturizer between your hands to soften it (if necessary) and apply to your face and neck.

*Although coconuts are not true nuts, if you have a nut allergy, please patch test this recipe first. I'm yet to see someone have a reaction, but you never know. A small dollop massaged into the inside of the wrist will tell you if you're fine with it topically. If not you can easily substitute coconut oil for cocoa butter or shea butter (slightly creamier, but still effective).

Aloe & Geranium Night Cream

Aloe vera is such an all-rounder: you can drink it, eat it and wear it. This recipe calls for the juice as opposed to the gel, but the benefits are just as potent. I love this moisturizer when my skin is stressed out and looks dry and patchy. Despite its thick creaminess, it's surprisingly non-oily and very restorative for problem skin (too much oil = blemishes).

  I recommend making this when you have time on your hands and don't mind making mess. For mothers of girls, this is the best cream to make with your teenage daughters: it's perfect for young skin and gives you time to be together. #girlpower

Makes about 300ml/10½fl oz/
    1 cup + 3 tbsp
Shelf life: 6 months

15g/½oz beeswax beads
30g/1oz shea butter
60ml/2fl oz/¼ cup kukui nut oil
185ml/6fl oz/¾ cup aloe vera juice
4 drops geranium essential oil
2 drops neroli essential oil
2 drops orange essential oil
½ tsp vitamin E oil or extra-virgin
    olive oil

Place a large saucepan of water on to boil. Once boiling, reduce the heat to low and allow to simmer. In a large, heatproof glass jar (you'll need one with a wide enough neck to fit a hand blender), add the beeswax, shea butter and kukui nut oil. Stand the jar in the saucepan of simmering water and allow the contents to melt together. Remove from the pan (take care, it will be hot) and set aside to cool.

Meanwhile, pour the aloe vera juice into another heatproof glass jar and allow this to heat in the saucepan of water in the same way.

Once the wax mixture is cool and has started turning milky, gently pour the aloe vera into the wax mixture little by little, using a stick blender to blend between each addition, If you can, blend as you add – this is where a helping hand is a good idea. The wax can't absorb all the liquid in one go, so keep adding and blending until the texture is creamy and the liquids no longer separate – be patient, it takes time, but it will happen!

When the mixture is beautifully creamy, stir in the essential oils and vitamin E or extra-virgin olive oil, then beat again – you should have a lovely, thick and creamy mixture. Pop the lid on the jar to store. A little goes a long way: to use, rub a little moisturizer between your hands to soften (if necessary) and apply to your face and neck.

*If you don't have a jar with a neck wide enough to fit a stick blender, you can melt the wax mixture and warm the aloe vera in a double boiler, then combine in the wax bowl and transfer to a jar to store.

Refreshing Eye Gel

The ingredients in this eye gel help to ease the symptoms of eye strain and tired eyes, as well as being thoroughly rejuvenating. Gentle chamomile is anti-inflammatory to help reduce puffiness; and fennel and rosemary clarify and refresh the skin, while evening primrose and aloe are champions when it comes to reducing wrinkles.

Makes about 80ml/2½fl oz/
  ⅓ cup
Shelf life: 3 months in the fridge

1 chamomile tea bag
½ tsp gelatine powder
1 tbsp aloe vera gel
2 tsp evening primrose oil
1 drop fennel essential oil
2 drops rosemary essential oil

Put the tea bag into a measuring jug and pour over 60ml/2fl oz/¼ cup boiling water. Leave to infuse for 5 minutes to make a strong brew. Remove the tea bag and then sprinkle in the gelatine, stirring until it dissolves. (If the tea has cooled too much to dissolve the gelatine, reheat it gently by placing the jug in a pan of hot water, but don't let it boil as this can impair the setting qualities of the gelatine.)

Once the gelatine has dissolved, add the remaining ingredients and whisk together with a balloon whisk until well incorporated. Place the jug in the fridge to set the mixture, stirring everything together a couple of times as it cools and sets. To use, dab a little gel on your fingertip and apply under and to the sides of your eyes, taking care not to get the gel actually in your eyes (if you do, just rinse with fresh water). This gel is particularly refreshing if you use it straight from the fridge.

Coconut & Rooibos Moisturizer

I'm a bit crazy about coconuts, especially as a moisturizer. Here, I combine them with rooibos (Afrikaans for 'redbush') tea, which is another one of those youth miracles, because it helps rehydrate skin, flush toxins, repair cells and refresh the complexion. If you want to maximize the shelf-life, omit the coconut milk powder.

Makes about 250ml/9fl oz/1 cup
Shelf life: 3 months

1 rooibos (redbush) teabag
2 tsp coconut milk powder
    (optional)
200ml/9fl oz/1 cup coconut oil
30g/1oz shea butter

First, make a strong tea infusion. Steep the teabag in 3 tbsp of boiling water in a small glass bowl for 15 minutes. Remove the tea bag from the infusion and stir in the coconut milk powder (if using), then set aside to cool.

While the tea is cooling, make a double boiler by placing a glass bowl over a pan of simmering water. Allow the water to lap at the bowl, but not to flow over the edges of the pan. Add the coconut oil and shea butter, allow to melt, then remove the bowl (take care – the bowl will be hot) and set aside to cool slightly until just soft set. Use a hand whisk to whip it up to a creamy texture (about 5 minutes), then add the tea a little at a time, whisking again between each addition, until you've used all the tea and you have a thick, fluffy mixture. Transfer to a cosmetics pot with a lid.

To use, rub just a little moisturizer between your hands to soften (if necessary) and apply to your face and neck.

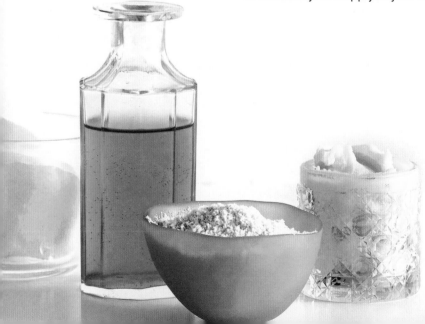

The 'Extra-care' Essentials

If you Google 'wardrobe basics' you'll get a list of clothing staples every woman (and man) should have ready to go. A complete mix-and-match list for the minimalists or those finally out of school uniforms. Everything else is just for fun or event specific. In skincare, the three-step system is your staple, but staples alone can get a little dull and sometimes your skin needs just a bit more. The following is a series of solutions for specific skin issues; some I recommend adopting into your skincare routine often, and others are optional for every now and then.

Personally, I like to incorporate some extras into my routine each week, particularly exfoliating and masking. I also use a serum every evening, after I've applied my moisturizer. As my skin takes a makeup beating, it tends to need much more care than I think it would if I worked in an office. We're all different and your skin will tell you what it likes, so have some fun experimenting with these and even think about doing your own DIY facial every so often.

SERUMS
(AKA THE GLOW ENHANCERS)
The purpose of a serum is to reach below the surface of the skin to the layers beneath. Serum ingredients are lipid-soluble, which means they penetrate deeply to correct issues in the skin that we can't see. A good serum should be loaded with antioxidants and nutrients specific to your skin.

MASKS
(AKA PURIFY AND PROTECT)
Applying a mask is a little like submerging your skin in a bathtub full of goodness. Because we tend to leave masks on for 15–20 minutes, they can penetrate to correct damage that lies deep. A good mask should perform for your individual skin type and concerns.

FACIALS
(AKA INDULGE AND PAMPER)
Put simply, a facial is just a combination of different steps from basics to extras, all in one go. It's like doing a detox for your skin. The order is really up to you, but my facials tend to go like this – cleanse, steam (face over a bowl of hot water with a towel covering the head), mask, exfoliate, tone, moisturize, serum. If you have an hour in which to do as you like, then I definitely recommend pampering your skin with one of these.

SCRUBS
(AKA BUFF AND RENEW)
A scrub is basically a gritty version of a cleanser. It's designed to remove debris, dead cells and unclog pores. The 'grit' is an exfoliator; something designed to really buff and polish the outer layer and allow for healthy cell regeneration.

SPOT CORRECTORS
(AKA BLEMISHES BE GONE)
Spot correctors are a fairly new invention, although if you ask your grandparents I'll guarantee they could rattle off a list of things they did for blemishes in their day. While there isn't a 'spot disappear' miracle cream, there are plenty of things that help. The best correctors are ones that not only assist the removal process but also heal the underlying tissue.

SERUMS
#makeitglow

It's a beauty misconception that serums are just a more expensive form of moisturizer. While they do work out a little pricier, you're actually getting a more concentrated product that can penetrate to a deeper level.

A serum is my go-to for improving the overall quality of my skin and achieving a healthy, youthful glow. The active ingredients can feed antioxidants to the skin, restore cell growth and help decrease pore size; in fact, the only thing they really don't do is moisturize. That's right, it's an extra not an all-rounder. Moisturizers have a base that allows them to stay on the surface to moisturize and protect the outer layer of your skin, but a serum is designed to penetrate the epidermis and reach the layers underneath.

Use a serum only at night as exposure to UV rays can cause the serum to oxidize, which can damage the cell structure of your skin. I personally use a serum each night after my moisturizer to deeply heal my skin while I sleep. Best of all, this means waking up in the morning with a beautiful, glowing complexion.

If you've got acne-prone skin and you're unsure whether a serum is for you, don't fear. Use ones containing retinol (found in dairy products) and/or vitamin C (in fruit and vegetables, such as avocado; see page 65) as both of these antioxidants improve cell growth and remove blemishes faster.

X

Serums
#everyonelovesaquickie

Rosehip Oil
THE ANTI-AGER

Rosehip oil has so much nutritional potential for your skin, it's hard to know where to start! It's rich in essential fatty acids to help strengthen and regenerate the walls of skin cells and is loaded with vitamin A, an important antioxidant that helps strengthen the collagen in the skin, improving elasticity and smoothing out fine lines. If you are worried about stretch marks, rosehip oil is essential for your #everyonelovesaquickie rescue bag – rub a few drops into the affected area every day just before bed for a month and watch those little tear-and-repairs melt away. You can take the same approach for beating laughter-lines, too.

Sea Buckthorn Oil
THE SUPERFOOD WARRIOR

Sea buckthorns are little orange berries found in coastal regions – they are loaded with antioxidants, such as vitamins C and E, and have a high concentration of essential fatty acids, altogether making this little-cherished fruit a warrior in wrinkle prevention. Use the oil on your face to smooth out wrinkles and strengthen elasticity, maintaining your youthful appearance. You can use it no matter what your skin type, and it's even great for those of us who are prone to blemishes. To use, gently massage a few drops into your skin and allow to soak in before going to bed.

Evening Primrose Oil
THE ACNE BLITZER

Evening primrose oil is a miracle-worker for your skin. It's loaded with omega-6 essential fatty acids, which help strengthen the skin-cell walls, reducing inflammation and maintaining a blemish-free complexion. For acne, evening primrose oil helps to balance out the effects of sebum, the skin's natural moisturizer, which when overproduced leads to those characteristic spots. To use, every day gently massage a few drops into the skin and allow to soak in before going to bed – you should see results in about 4 weeks.

Carrot Seed Oil
THE 'ALL-ROUND' HEALER

Is there anything this oil can't do? It works for all skin types and all conditions, no exceptions, which makes it the perfect choice if you have especially sensitive skin. The oil contains such an abundance of nutrients that some claim it to be the most heavy-duty, all-purpose healing oil in the world. It's main constituent is the antioxidant beta-carotene (the precursor to vitamin A). It's one of the few oils with a natural sun protection factor (SPF), so as well as nourishing and rejuvenating the skin, it helps to protect it from UV light. Just one word of safety: unlike the other #quickies on this page, carrot seed is an essential oil and needs to be diluted in a carrier oil before you apply it to your skin. So, to use it, dilute 1 drop of carrot seed essential oil in 1 tsp of extra-virgin olive oil and gently massage the mixture into your skin. Allow it to soak in before going to bed.

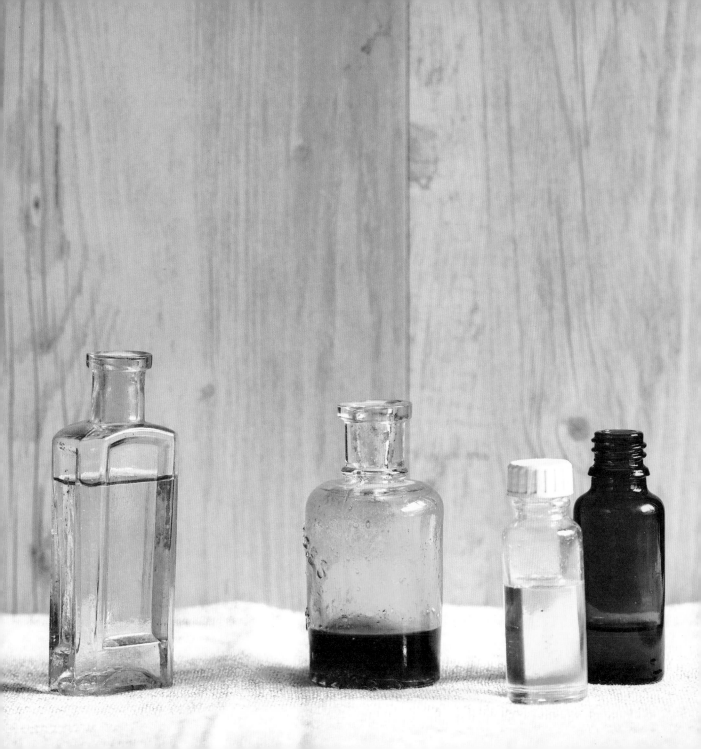

Rejuvenating Rosehip Serum

Up until now, this has been one of my best-kept beauty secrets – and I'm so excited to share it with you. If you've ever read a magazine then you're probably all too aware of a special application called Photoshop: it's that handy bit of technology that removes imperfections in the blink of an eye (or rather the press of a button). What you probably didn't know is that it's expensive, and I mean *CRAZY* expensive – in some cases retouching can cost a thousand dollars a minute. There's a reason models are starting to get serious about their skin and why casting directors will make you take off your makeup if you're wearing it at a go-see (model audition). The girls with the best skin are the girls getting booked, so flawless, glowing skin is a must. The night before a casting or a shoot I lather (and yes I'm talking several layers) my face in this serum. In the morning my skin looks like a photograph that could grace the cover of *Vogue* – and this is sans makeup.

Makes about 15ml/½fl oz/1 tbsp
Shelf life: 3 months

2 tsp hemp seed oil
1 tsp rosehip oil
2 drops frankincense essential oil
2 drops rose geranium essential oil

Measure the oils into a small, dark-glass bottle. Place the cap on the bottle, secure, and shake to combine. To use, warm a little serum in the palms of your hands and smooth over your face and neck.

Avocado & Rose Acne Healing Serum

I love this serum if I'm having trouble with my skin – it not only helps to reduce breakouts, but can also help to reduce acne scarring (if like me, you've struggled with the problem since high school). There's nothing so shattering to your confidence than having acne, but harsh, 'cure-acne' products that supposedly strip oils are actually doing far more damage to your skin than good.

This combination of oils assists the body in regulating the hormones that cause blemishes and over-production of sebum. They work on a cellular level and are restorative as well as corrective. Try not to get too overexcited and apply this every 5 minutes; once an evening is plenty and it can do all the hard work while you sleep.

Makes about 15ml/½fl oz/1 tbsp
Shelf life: 3 months

1½ tsp avocado oil
½ tsp vitamin E oil
1 tsp calendula oil
15 drops rose geranium essential oil
15 drops orange leaf essential oil

Combine all the oils in a small, dark-glass bottle. Place the cap on the bottle, secure, and shake to combine. To use, warm a little serum in the palms of your hands and smooth over your face, neck and upper chest.

*Calendula, rose geranium and orange leaf oils are great for clearing and balancing sebum levels and excess oils in acne-prone skin.

SPOT CORRECTORS
#blemishbusters

Blemish (n): a small mark or flaw that spoils the appearance of something.

In an ideal world we would all be born with flawless skin, our hormones would never go out of whack, and we'd never produce excess oil and end the day shiny enough to cook an egg on our face. But sadly it's not an ideal world and blemishes are a fact for everyone and every skin type – at every age. I had problem skin during almost all of high school and it was gutting. I was so self-conscious I quite often had a fringe just to keep my spots covered (honestly, if I could have gotten away with it, I would have worn a paper bag over my head). There were girls whose skin was perfect and equally as many girls who were always being sent to remove their makeup because they had troubles like me.

To bust a common myth, acne has very little to do with oil and almost everything to do with hormones, which is why it tends to affect teenagers more than adults. There are countless products that are marketed to the 'blemish bunch' with the amazing promises of clearing skin for good. Don't misunderstand me, they work. They are loaded with stripping agents that pull excess oil and impurities from the top layer. Problem is, you have to use them for ever, and in 10 years you'll look 20 years older.

I'm all too aware that aging isn't something a young person thinks about, but if you knew at 15 that the products curing your pimples would make you appear 35 at the age of 25, I'm sure you would think twice. Oily, acne-prone, blackhead-infested skin still needs nourishing: there are no exceptions and the right three-step system designed for you will do exactly that (while balancing the hormones that cause all those irritating problems).

If you're impatient (like me), then you want something you can do immediately to get rid of that spot that's decided your face is its new home. These recipes are all for busting those blemishes: everything from removing the dirt inside the spot, to reducing swelling and inflammation so it's not quite so unsightly.

Even now, I'm not immune to the odd breakout (particularly when I'm stressed), so I keep a little arsenal of busters with me everywhere I go.

X

Blemish Busters
#everyonelovesaquickie

Each of these 'busters' will purify, heal and remove blemishes. They all unclog the pores, dry excess oil and are anti-inflammatory to reduce infection and swelling.

Aloe Vera & Cucumber

Cut, peel, deseed and blend a 2.5cm/1in piece of cucumber. Mix in 2 tbsp of aloe vera gel and 2 drops of tea tree oil. Apply and allow to dry before rinsing.

Apple Cider Vinegar

Dip a cotton bud in the vinegar and apply directly to blemishes. Rinse completely.

Aspirin & Lemon

Crush 6–12 non-coated aspirin and mix with just enough lemon juice to form a paste (it can take 5–10 minutes to thicken up, so be patient), then apply to your face. Leave for 5 minutes, then rinse thoroughly.

Banana & Yogurt

Mash 1 banana with 2 tbsp of natural yogurt. Apply to your face as a mask. Leave on for 2 hours, then rinse off.

Calamine & Lavender

Mix 3 tbsp of calamine lotion with 2 drops of lavender essential oil. Apply to the whole face, leave in place for 3–4 hours, then rinse off.

Ginger Root

Cut a 2.5cm/1in piece of fresh ginger, peel and rub it all over your face. Leave for 5 minutes, then rinse. You can combine grated ginger with a little honey and oatmeal to create a mask, if you prefer.

Lemon & Bicarb

Cut a wedge of lemon and squeeze the juice into a tablespoon of bicarbonate of soda (baking soda) until you have a thick paste. Use a cotton wool pad to cover blackheads, leave for 10 minutes and rinse off.

Honey & Cinnamon

Put a pinch of cinnamon in a teaspoon of honey and use a cotton bud to dab directly on blemishes.

Orange Peel & Rose Water

Grate and combine the peel of 1 orange with 1 tbsp of natural yogurt and 1 tbsp of rose water. Apply to the face as a mask; leave for 1 hour, then rinse off.

Sandalwood & Turmeric

Mix 1 tbsp of sandalwood with ½ tbsp of turmeric powder, then add natural yogurt to form a thick paste. Loosen slightly with a squeeze of lemon juice. Apply to the face and leave for 3–4 hours, then rinse off.

---

*Bathe face in *BUTTERMILK* to reduce swelling.

*Apply *COCONUT OIL* to fade scars.

*Wash daily with cold, brewed *GREEN TEA* to purify.

*Wash daily with *ROSE WATER* to calm rosacea.

*For blackheads, mix 1 tbsp of gelatine and 1½ tbsp of milk. Form a paste, apply, allow to dry, then rinse.

*Wrap an *ICE CUBE* in a tissue and hold it on a spot for 30 seconds to reduce swelling and anaesthetize.

ALCOHOL applied with a cotton bud (post squeeze) is a natural disinfectant to protect against spread.

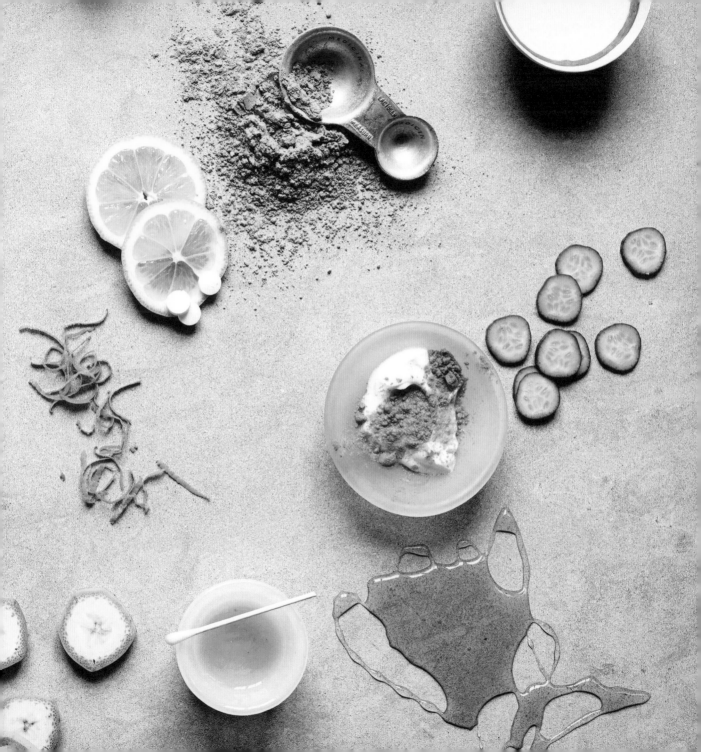

Protective Burdock Skin-repair Lotion

I like to use this as a spot treatment, but you can use it in place of a moisturizer if your skin is really problematic. It contains burdock root, which is wonderful for reducing inflammation and drawing toxins out of your skin. It also harbours a little powdery mineral called zinc oxide; you may have heard of it as it's the main ingredient in most sunscreens, because – even though it sounds like something that you'd use to galvanize a nail – it is one of the safest completely natural ingredients for protecting the skin from UV rays and repairing skin cells. It's also amazing for acne as it creates a strong barrier against external irritants that can cause breakouts all of their own.

If you're using this recipe as a spot treatment, just dab a little on the affected area using a cotton bud, and let it dry.

Makes about 150ml/5fl oz/
    scant ⅔ cup
Shelf life: 2 months in the fridge

2 tbsp avocado oil
15g/½oz shea butter
5g/⅛oz soy wax
5g/⅛oz emulsifying wax
1 tbsp burdock root tea
1 tsp liquid vegetable glycerine
1 tsp zinc oxide
4 drops elemi essential oil
3 drops tangerine essential oil
3 drops tea tree essential oil
2 drops fennel essential oil

Make a double boiler by placing a glass bowl over a pan of simmering water. Allow the water to lap at the bowl, but not to flow over the edges of the pan. Add the avocado oil, shea butter and waxes and allow to melt, then remove the bowl (take care – the bowl will be hot) and allow to cool slightly.

Meanwhile, put the tea in a jug and pour over 100ml/3½fl oz/⅓ cup + 2 tbsp of boiling water. Allow to infuse for 10 minutes, then strain the liquid and discard the used tea (you can use a tea infuser if you have one). Stir in the vegetable glycerine, zinc oxide and essential oils – you need to do this while the tea is still warm, so that the wax doesn't start to solidify as soon as you bring the two mixtures together in the next step.

Once the wax mixture has started to solidify and turn milky, whip it up with a hand whisk until thick and creamy. Once you've reached the right consistency, very slowly add the infusion mixture – just little by little – whisking well between each addition. When all the infusion is fully combined, keep whisking until the mixture has cooled and formed a lotion. Transfer to a cosmetics pot and store in the fridge.

*You don't always have to put these lotions and potions in pots. You can use lotion tubes, which you'll find at most chemists or department stores (just ask for their travel tubes). For gifts, though, little glass jars look so beautiful.

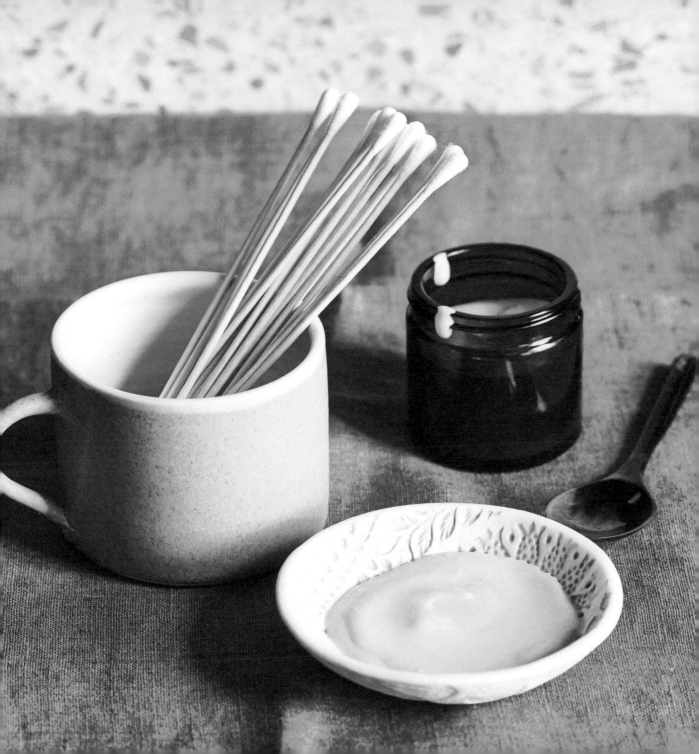

Cinnamon Anti-Blackhead Mask

When a pore gets so blocked up it can't take any more, it seals itself away from the world and goes into lockdown. The result is what looks like a little black spot on your skin. Use this beauty staple to open up your pores again, clear away the impurities and restore your complexion to blemish-free status.

Makes about 30ml/1fl oz/2 tbsp
Shelf life: 1–2 weeks in the fridge, but best used immediately

1 tsp ground cinnamon
1 tsp bicarbonate of soda (baking soda)
½ tsp kaolin clay

Put the cinnamon, bicarbonate of soda and kaolin clay in a small glass bowl or cup and stir to combine. Then, very slowly (drop by drop if you can – a pipette is a good idea, or use a sterilized teaspoon) add fresh water, mixing between each addition until you have formed a paste.

To use, apply the paste to the affected area, over the blackheads, and leave in place for 15–20 minutes. Rinse off with fresh water, then cleanse, tone and moisturize your skin.

*Cinnamon has powerful antibacterial properties, helping to rid your skin of the locked-in impurities, and bicarbonate of soda gently exfoliates to open up the pores.

Carbon & Yogurt Spot Healer

Makes about 70ml/2¼fl oz/
    scant ⅓ cup
Shelf life: use immediately

1 tbsp bentonite clay (see safety
    note on page 28)
1 tbsp arrowroot powder
½ tbsp activated charcoal
1 aspirin tablet, ground to a fine
    powder
1 tbsp natural yogurt
1 tbsp aloe vera gel
3 drops tea tree essential oil
3 drops myrtle essential oil
1 drop frankincense essential oil

Whenever I think about carbon, I am immediately transported back to lazy Sunday afternoons watching my dad load charcoal into the BBQ (pretty standard if you grow up in Australia). If you'd told me on one of those occasions that I'd one day be using that disgusting dirt on my face (and recommending it no less), I probably would have slapped you. However, carbon (or in this case charcoal – which is in fact the dehydrogenated residue from carbon and ash) boasts some serious beauty benefits. This recipe contains not the debris from Sunday's grilled steak, but 'activated charcoal', which is carbon that has been treated with oxygen. It draws out bacteria, toxins, dirt and other tiny particles from the skin in proportions thousands of times greater than its own mass.

Aspirin is actually a remedy my grandmother taught me for helping clear up my problem skin. It's an anti-inflammatory and contains some of the same ingredients as white willow bark, which is why they're often used together to treat really bad acne. Aspirin can unclog pores (of anything, not just dirt, so it's also great for ingrown hairs), reduce swelling and even soften your skin. While I tend to use herbal remedies for curing ailments, I do always have a bottle of aspirin in my kitchen to use whenever I need to bust a blemish.

Place all the ingredients in a small, glass bowl (remember bentonite must not come into contact with metal – so you must use a glass bowl!) and stir thoroughly with a wooden or plastic spoon to combine.

To use, apply to your face and leave for 15–20 minutes. Rinse with fresh water, then cleanse, tone and moisturize.

FACE SCRUBS

#inthebuff

If you've ever been to Australia, then you'll understand the obsession we Australians have with beaches. They are not just a part of our geography, or even our culture, they are a part of who we are. Summer or winter, day or night, there's never a bad time to hit the waves and while I might be a little biased, our beaches are really quite magical. They're also good for your health (and your beauty routine). Ever noticed how unbelievably 'hot' you look after a day in the surf? It's the reason so many brands produce things like textured sea spray to create hair that looks like you've stepped out of the ocean, bronzers to give that sun-kissed beach glow and sea minerals to promote radiant skin.

I need to share a little secret with you – I have terrible feet. Yep, cracked, flaky, damaged, and this is before I start on the bone problems from years of wearing pointe shoes. Now, if you told me I never had to wear shoes a day in my life, I would be ecstatic. I love the feel of the ground beneath my feet and when I'm travelling the first thing I do in a new place is take off my shoes and feel the earth... I'm a barefoot baby! Being barefoot isn't great for your soles, though, as on most surfaces it hardens and dries out the skin, but spend a day walking on the sand and your feet are good as new – being a beach baby has its skin benefits.

Basically, the sand acts as an exfoliator, and exfoliation is one of the most amazing things you can do to refresh and regenerate your skin. If you've come this far, then you know cleansing is a must, but a twice-weekly scrub with something a little grittier can completely transform your skin. It removes any dead cells, unclogs all the pores, tightens and tones the connective tissue and can reduce the signs of aging. I personally use a scrub from my face to my feet a few times each week to keep my skin looking and feeling its best. This might be an extra, but it's definitely worth the investment.

X

Face Scrubs
#everyonelovesaquickie

The following list is a mix-and-match guide. Most homemade scrubs are really easy to make, but if you want a 'no-brainer' just choose an exfoliant and a liquid from each list and you're good to go. To use, mix 1 tsp of exfoliant with 1 tbsp of liquid, then apply to the face and rinse. Easy peasy!

EXFOLIANTS

Oily Skin The ingredients in this list are the most gritty, so if you have super-oily skin, these are for you.
- Macrobiotic Sea Salt (or you can use ordinary sea salt)
- Granulated Raw Sugar
- Organic Brown Rice

Dry Skin These ingredients are a little more nourishing to protect against cell damage as well as remove debris.
- Organic Ground Coffee
- Sunflower Seeds
- Apricot Kernels

Sensitive Skin As sensitive skin is prone to capillary damage, these are the most mild and gentle scrubs.
- Almond Meal (Ground Almonds)
- Organic Oats
- Natural Yogurt (this doesn't require a liquid)

LIQUIDS

Oily Skin These ingredients dissolve excess oil so are the best to use if you have oily skin.
- Extra-virgin Olive Oil
- Macadamia Nut Oil
- Lemon Juice

Dry Skin These ingredients have more moisture in them, which helps to protect against flaking skin.
- Coconut Oil
- Jojoba Oil
- Sunflower Oil

Sensitive Skin These ingredients are the most gentle and nourishing, so they're perfect for sensitive and older skin.
- Full-fat Milk
- Sweet Almond Oil
- Filtered Water

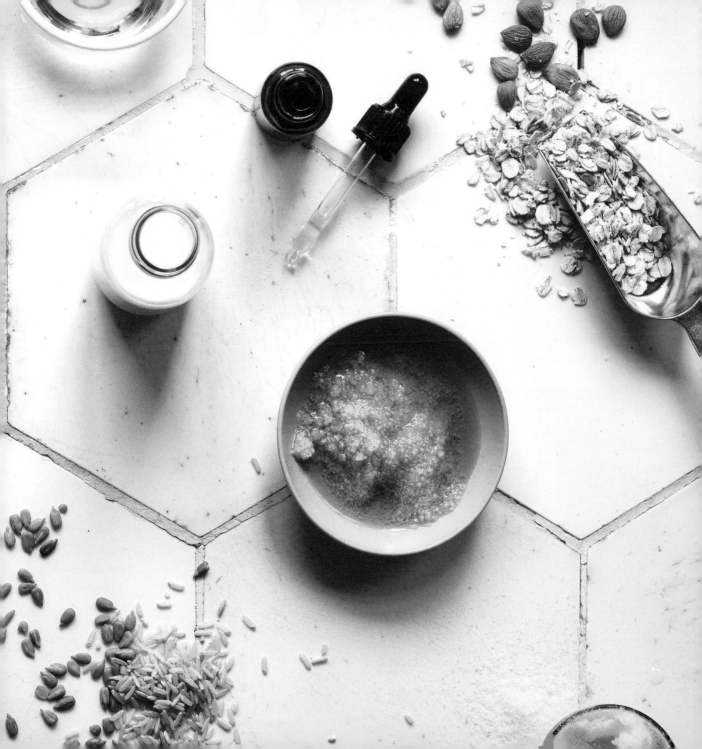

Kiwi & Avocado Face Scrub

Kiwis are loaded with nutrients – in particular vitamin C, which when applied topically to the skin is great for restoring a tired complexion and giving the skin a healthy glow. Add to that the vitamin E and essential fats in avocado, and your face will radiate pure love.

Makes about 60ml/2fl oz/¼ cup
Shelf life: Use immediately

½ kiwi fruit, peeled
¼ avocado
1 tsp lemon or lime juice
¼ tsp jojoba oil
2½ tbsp fine salt crystals

Place the kiwi flesh in a blender along with the flesh from the half avocado. Pulse to mulch everything together – it doesn't matter if there are a few lumps left over – a full purée can go too runny. Tip the kiwi and avocado mixture into a bowl and stir in the lemon or lime juice, jojoba oil and salt crystals. Keep stirring until the salt crystals are evenly distributed. Apply immediately to your face, rubbing gently so that the crystals exfoliate your skin. Leave in place for 15–20 minutes, then rinse off and moisturize straightaway.

---

*For a longer-lasting version, you could omit the fresh avocado and replace it with another kiwi half and 1 tsp of avocado oil. This will store in an airtight container for up to 2 weeks.

*Always use fine salt crystals for a face scrub. If you want a deeper exfoliation on the soles of your feet, say, you can use a coarser salt, but coarse salt can cause microscopic skin tears on soft skin.

Honey & Oatmeal Blemish Scrub

This is my go-to scrub and, as I have quite sensitive skin, I find it the most effective one to use on a regular basis. Oats make a good exfoliant because they aren't too harsh on the skin, while the tea tree oil is great for blemishes. If you have severe acne or other skin conditions, then this is perfect for you: it's nourishing, but also antiseptic and a good all-around healer.

Makes about 150g/5½oz
Shelf life (before adding yogurt):
  6 weeks

100g/3½oz/½ cup organic oats
2 tbsp raw runny honey
1 tsp freshly grated nutmeg
15 drops tea tree oil
15 drops lavender essential oil

For each application:
1 tsp natural yogurt

Run the oats through a food processor to break them up into a coarse powder (about 20 seconds should do it – much longer and it will turn to oat dust). Add the honey, nutmeg, tea tree oil and lavender oil and briefly blend again to combine, then transfer to an airtight container to store.

To use, run a facecloth under warm water, then wring it out so that it is just damp. Use it to wet your face all over. Scoop out 1 tbsp of the oatmeal and combine this with 1 tsp natural yogurt. Massage the mixture into the skin on your face, avoiding your eyes. Leave for 5 minutes, then rinse and moisturize straightaway.

Hydrating Cucumber Face Scrub

After a busy period at work I'll quite often spend a good 2 weeks with this scrub as the richly skin-nourishing avocado and walnut oils make it highly restorative for a face that has been pounded with lots of makeup. Cucumber is incredibly hydrating for your skin, which makes it great for reducing inflammation and puffiness: it encourages thirsty skin cells to release the water they're holding on to. Whatever your skin type, this scrub will nourish, hydrate and soothe.

Makes about 350ml/12fl oz/
    1½ cups
Shelf life: 2 months in the fridge

¼ cucumber, halved lengthways
    and seeds removed
1 small handful mint, leaves picked
    and torn
250g/9oz granulated sugar
1 tbsp avocado oil
1 tbsp walnut oil
½ tbsp natural yogurt (optional)

Place the cucumber flesh (with the skin on) and the torn mint leaves into a bowl, then use a hand-held blender to pulse into a chunky purée (be careful not to break down the cucumber completely – it needs to be chunky rather than liquid; you can use a mini-processor if you prefer).

In a separate bowl mix the sugar, oils, and natural yogurt (if using). Spoon in the mint and cucumber mixture and stir to combine thoroughly. Transfer the scrub to a cosmetics jar (a Kilner jar with an airtight lid is ideal) and refrigerate until you need it. Mix well before each use.

To use, run a facecloth under warm water, then wring it out so that it is just damp. Use it to wet your face all over. Then, use your fingers to scoop out a little of the scrub (just a tablespoon should do it) and massage it into the skin on your face, avoiding your eyes. Leave the scrub on for 5–10 minutes, then rinse, and moisturize straightaway.

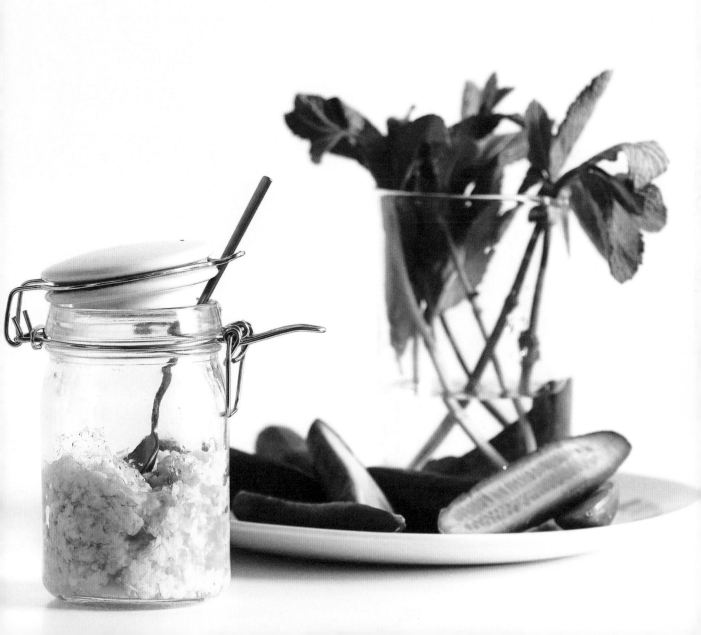

FACE MASKS
#mondaymaskandmultitask

I love masking and if you've ever had a facial (or a girls' slumber party) you know a mask can be extremely fun…. But do you know what a mask is for? It has always been one of my firm beliefs that before you smear something all over your face, you should know why you're doing it. Masks can, and do, do a lot of things! Depending on the ingredients, they can add moisture, remove oil, tighten pores, exfoliate, reduce puffiness and even help reduce signs of aging (not to mention they feel great).

Ever heard the line, 'I just want to go home, kick off my shoes and soak in a bath'? It's usually how you feel after a long day (or week) when your body is exhausted and needs not just relaxing but pampering; well a mask is exactly that. Your skin is working 24 hours a day repairing itself, rebuilding and growing cells, healing wounds or blemishes and expanding and contracting its structure. It never takes a break, not even for a second. Masking is like a bath for your skin; it allows you to combat specific issues, as well as offering all-round cleanliness, and gives your overworked cells a much-needed rest and dose of essential nutrients.

As part of my skincare routine, I mask twice a week with two different types. On Wednesdays I use a purifying clay mask for a deeper, more concentrated clean; and on Sundays I use a hydrating mask with moisturizing ingredients to relax, soften and renew my tired skin. If you're wearing makeup on a regular basis, I would recommend that you go for twice-weekly masking, too – although once a week is better than no mask at all.

Trial and error is really the best way to find exactly what works for you. When you've rinsed, your skin should be soft, smooth, glowing and rejuvenated. Have some fun with these recipes and mix and match until you've found the perfect combination.

X

Face Masks
#everyonelovesaquickie

From Your Fridge to Your Face

Each of these masks has a different benefit and all can be made using ingredients straight from your fridge. These masks are healing and corrective and just what the (skin) doctor ordered. Apply after cleansing.

Strawberries
COMBATS OIL

Mash a good handful and apply directly to the skin. Leave for 5–10 minutes, then rinse.

Avocado
PURIFIES AND HYDRATES

Mash half an avocado and a dash of lemon juice. Apply evenly and rinse after 10 minutes.

Eggs
TIGHTENS PORES

Whisk 2–3 egg whites and apply evenly. Leave for 15 minutes, then rinse.

Yogurt
LIGHTENS COMPLEXION

Apply 1 tbsp of natural yogurt directly to the skin and rinse after 10 minutes.

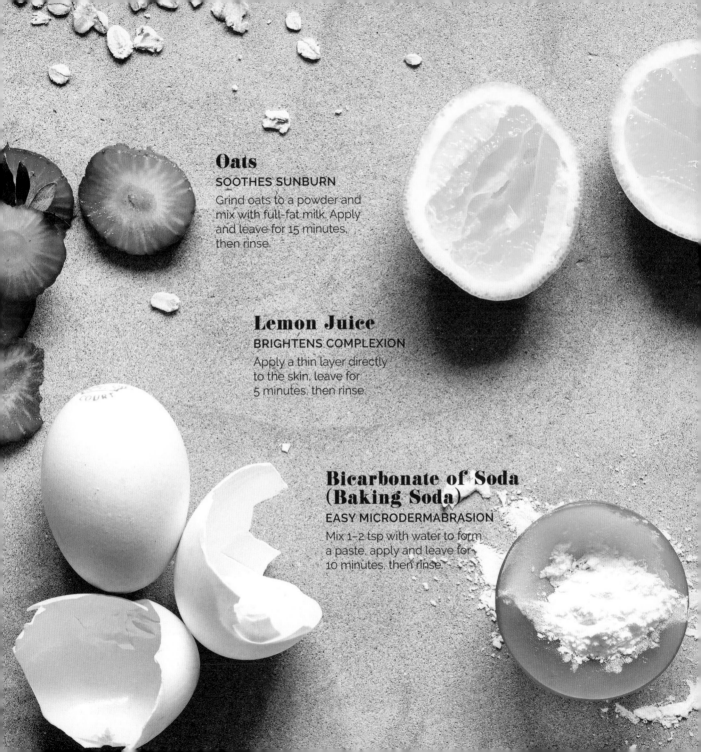

Oats

SOOTHES SUNBURN

Grind oats to a powder and mix with full-fat milk. Apply and leave for 15 minutes, then rinse.

Lemon Juice

BRIGHTENS COMPLEXION

Apply a thin layer directly to the skin, leave for 5 minutes, then rinse.

Bicarbonate of Soda (Baking Soda)

EASY MICRODERMABRASION

Mix 1–2 tsp with water to form a paste, apply and leave for 10 minutes, then rinse.

Complete Purifying Clay Mask

Meet my Wednesday mask: the ultimate deep clean, working hard to remove impurities. I love how fresh my skin feels after this and I can still feel the results several days later. It's not just a blemish-buster, but soothes and refines the skin, plus the honey gives it antiseptic properties to remove any germs or bacteria and stop the spread of blemishes and imperfections. It's particularly good if you have oily skin.

Makes about 40ml/1¼fl oz
Shelf life: use immediately

1 tbsp bentonite clay (see safety
   note on page 28)
1 tsp raw honey
3 drops essential oil of choice

Making this skin mask couldn't be easier. Mix all the ingredients together with 1 tbsp of filtered water in a small, non-metallic bowl using a wooden or plastic spoon (this is important as you are using bentonite clay).

To use, run a facecloth under warm water, then wring it out so that it is just damp. Use it to wet your face all over. Then, use your fingers to scoop out a little of the mask at a time, and apply to your skin evenly. Leave the mask in place for 15 minutes, rinse, then moisturize straightaway.

Clay & Walnut Pore-relief Mask

If, like me, you barely have a day when you go out without at least a basic covering on your face, you'll know that after a week of caking, your pores are left gasping for air. This clay mask works into the pores encouraging them to spit out the leftover nasties and breathe again, while the walnut oil replenishes and restores balance.

Makes about 100ml/3½fl oz/
⅓ cup + 2 tbsp
Shelf life: 2 weeks

4 tbsp kaolin clay
2 tbsp titanium dioxide powder
3 drops geranium essential oil
2 drops neroli essential oil
2 tsp walnut oil

Mix together the clay and titanium dioxide (see note below) in a small, glass bowl, then add the essential oils and walnut oil and stir to combine thoroughly. Then, little by little (a trickle at a time is fine), add once-boiled cooled water, stirring between each addition, until you have a thick, spreadable paste. Store in an airtight container in a cool, dark place.

To use, run a facecloth under warm water, then wring it out so that it is just damp. Use it to wet your face all over. Then, use your fingers to scoop out a little of the mask at a time, and apply to your skin evenly. Leave for 15 minutes, rinse, then moisturize straightaway.

*If you already have zinc oxide in your cupboard, you can use this in place of the titanium dioxide powder. The results are similar and I'm all for saving on cost and minimizing waste.

Date & Pumpkin Face Mask

Vegetables that contain high amounts of vitamin C, carotenoids and zinc are not only nutritional superstars, but they provide the perfect base for a face mask, too. In this one, dates provide zinc and vitamins C and D to help minimize the signs of aging and improve skin elasticity. Any orange vegetable is packed with beta-carotene and vitamin C, so in this case the carrot and pumpkin give a double whammy. Finally, the cinnamon or nutmeg provides gentle exfoliation and helps unblock those toxin-laden pores.

Makes about 45ml/1½fl oz
Shelf life: 3 days in the fridge, but best used immediately

3 dates
2 tbsp pumpkin purée
1 tsp carrot juice
1 tsp raw honey
¼ tsp ground cinnamon or nutmeg

Soak the dates in hot water for 10 minutes to soften, then discard the soaking water. Put the dates in a mini-processor and blitz to a paste (or use a hand-held blender). Add the remaining ingredients and blitz again to fully combine and create a thick, smooth mask.

To use, run a facecloth under warm water, then wring it out so that it is just damp. Use it to wet your face all over. Then, use your fingers to scoop out a little of the mask at a time and apply to your skin evenly. Leave in place for 10–15 minutes, then rinse thoroughly with warm water and moisturize straightaway.

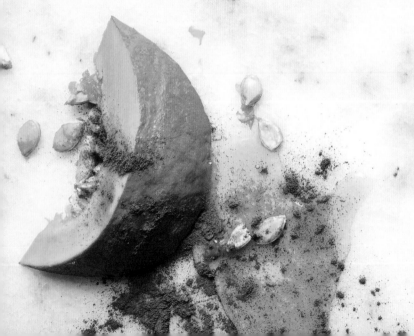

Watermelon & Avocado Super-hydrating Skin Mask

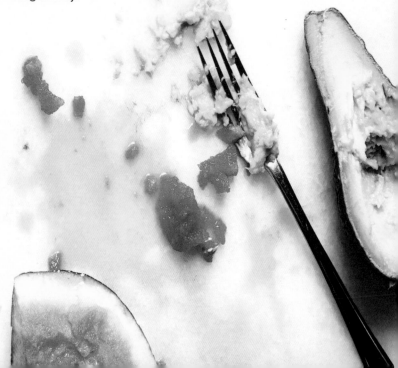

Makes about 70ml/2¼fl oz/
scant ⅓ cup
Shelf life: use immediately

1 tbsp raw honey
15g/½oz coconut oil
50g/2oz watermelon, pips
  removed
½ avocado, peeled and flesh
  chopped
5 drops tangerine essential oil

This is one of my favourite Sunday masks to really nourish the skin with vitamins and antioxidants before the week ahead. It's hydrating and rejuvenating if your skin is lacking lustre and looking run down.

Set a small glass bowl over a saucepan of gently simmering water. Add the honey and coconut oil. Warm them through until they become liquid – but don't let them get too hot! Remove the bowl from the pan and leave them to cool, but not so that they re-solidify.

Slice the melon flesh away from the skin and cut it into small pieces. Place the melon pieces with the honey, coconut oil and the remaining ingredients in a food processor and blend until you have a smooth paste.

To use, run a facecloth under warm water, then wring it out so that it is just damp. Use it to wet your face all over. Then, use your fingers to scoop out a little of the mask at a time and apply to your skin evenly. Leave for 30–35 minutes, then rinse thoroughly with warm water and moisturize straightaway.

PERFECT BASE
#foundationforgreatness

Okay, so we know all the reasons why wearing makeup is disastrous for your skin – it dries it out, clogs it up and in the end brings out more blemishes than it tries to conceal (I see a vicious cycle emerging). And there's no doubt that most shop-bought makeup bases contain nasties that really do nothing for your skin health. However, if you can create a makeup base that is kind and nourishing to your skin, while evening out appearance and making you feel ready to face the world, then perhaps it's not all bad. From foundations to bronzers, I'm happy to say that it's all possible.

Makeup should be fun, and in my opinion, restorative. These recipes are designed to replenish and rejuvenate the skin, correct imperfections and boost cell renewal, all while giving you an even-toned, glowing complexion.

X

PS Unfortunately, there's no real #everyonelovesaquickie for foundation, but if you mix a little powder that matches your complexion with your moisturizer then you've got something that'll work at a pinch.

Cocoa Butter Liquid Foundation

I rarely wear foundation outside of work, mostly because I'm lazy, but sometimes I have an event or product launch that requires a little extra effort on my part.

   The list of ingredients for this foundation is quite long, but it's so easy to make and it provides essential nutrients to repair the skin all while keeping you 'covered'. I love the magic when you start adding the colour.

Makes about 115ml/3¾fl oz/
   scant ½ cup
Shelf life: 3 months

20g/½oz soy wax
20g/½oz mango butter
20g/½oz cocoa butter
50ml/1½fl oz kukui nut oil
¼ tsp avocado oil
Pinch of ground cinnamon,
   plus extra for colour-matching
   if needed
1 tbsp cornflour (cornstarch) or
   arrowroot powder
Cocoa powder (amount will vary
   according to the colour of your
   skin)

Make a double boiler by placing a glass bowl over a pan of simmering water. Allow the water to lap at the bowl, but not to flow over the edges of the pan. Add the soy wax, mango and cocoa butters and both oils, and allow to melt, stirring occasionally to help them along the way. Remove the bowl from the pan (take care – the bowl will be hot) and set aside to cool slightly, but not so that the mixture re-solidifies. Use a hand mixer to beat the wax, butter and oil mixture until it is fully combined and you have a creamy consistency, about 3–5 minutes. Stir in the pinch of cinnamon.

Now comes the alchemy. Slowly start to add the powders, starting with the cornstarch or arrowroot powder. Stir this through, then add just a pinch of cocoa powder. Stir again. If it looks about right at this point, test a little on the back of your hand. If it's still too light, add another pinch of cocoa, stir and test again. Keep going like this until you get a good match. You'll find you can probably go a little darker than your natural skin colour, as the foundation goes on lighter than the mixture appears. However, if you go too far, add a pinch more cornflour or arrowroot (but see note below), and if you need it bronzed a little, add an extra pinch of cinnamon. When you're happy, spoon the foundation into an airtight cosmetics pot and use as needed.

*It's really hard to come back from a cream that is too dark, so be patient – if you add too much cocoa powder, you're likely to have to start again.

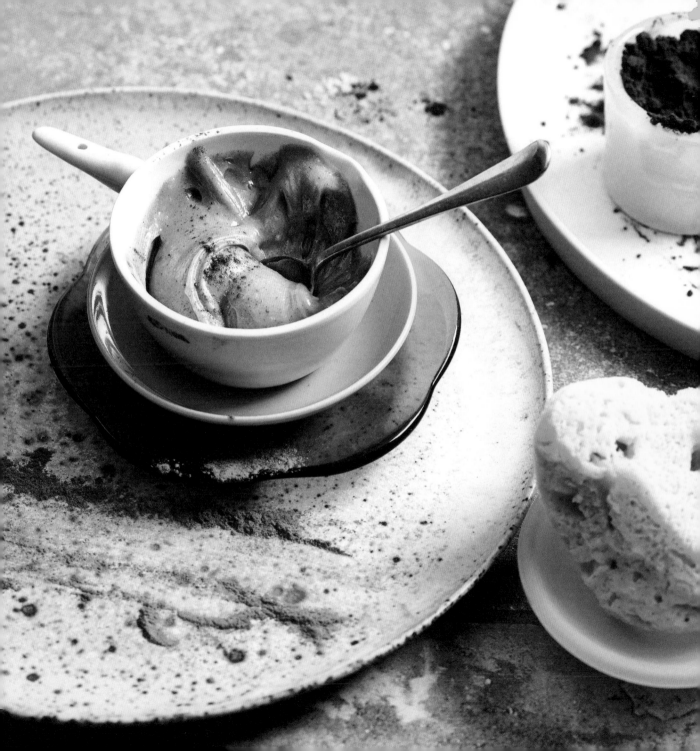

Perfect Clay Concealer

Concealer is one of those didn't-know-it-was-there products makeup artists have been using for decades. If you've got dark circles, uneven skin tone, blemishes or just a tired complexion, then this is a must in your arsenal. I tend to be a terrible sleeper and changing time zones does not help, so I rely on this one a lot when I'm working for the black baggies that form under my eyes. It's also corrective, so it heals blemishes at the same time as covering them (instead of making them worse).

Makes about 50g/2oz
Shelf life: 3 months

5g/⅛oz beeswax
5g/⅛oz shea butter
10g/¼oz cocoa butter
1 tsp macadamia nut oil
3 drops marula oil
1 tsp zinc oxide, plus extra for
    colour-matching
¾ tsp untreated sericite mica
2 tbsp kaolin clay
Brown, black, yellow and red
    iron oxides
Orchid ultramarine powder
Green mica powder

To conceal dark circles:
Add an extra pinch of yellow iron
    oxide if you have fair skin, or of
    orchid ultramarine powder if you
    have dark skin

To conceal blemishes:
Add an extra pinch of green
    mica powder or brown iron oxide

Make a double boiler by placing a glass bowl over a pan of simmering water. Allow the water to lap at the bowl, but not to flow over the edges of the pan. Add the three butters and the macadamia nut oil. Allow everything to melt together, then stir to combine. Remove the bowl from the pan (take care – the bowl will be hot) and set aside to cool slightly, but not so that the mixture re-solidifies. Add the marula oil, then use a hand mixer to beat the mixture until it is fully combined and you have a creamy consistency, about 3–5 minutes. Beat in the zinc oxide, sericite mica and kaolin clay until you achieve an even, creamy base colour.

Using the tips on colour-matching in the note below, very patiently mix in the oxides. Aim for a skin-tone match first, testing on the back of your hand between each addition until you're happy. Then, because this is a concealer, aim for a little darker, warmer or cooler, depending upon your need – for dark circles, you need to go a little warmer; for blemishes, a little cooler or darker. Experiment until you have something that conceals and then 'disappears' once you cover it with foundation and/or face powder. Practice makes perfect with this, so don't give up – keep trying and testing until you're happy. To use, apply as you would any shop-bought concealer.

*Zinc oxide will give your concealer a white base colour, so you'll need iron oxides to turn that into skin tone. Pinch by pinch mix in yellow, brown and red iron oxides until you get the right colour to match your skin. Keep a note of each addition, so that you can easily refer back to what worked (or didn't!). If you go too dark, use a little extra zinc oxide to lighten up again; if you need to go darker (rather than necessarily 'warmer'), add a little black iron oxide.

Gentle Translucent Face Powder

A powder is usually used to 'set' the foundation and give it a matte finish that looks more natural. Sometimes I use a powder by itself just to give my face a little colour (as I tend to look peaky) and this recipe makes a great version that I can use on its own – the oils give it just enough stickability.

Makes about 40g/1½oz
Shelf life: 6 months

3 tbsp arrowroot powder, plus extra for colour-matching
2 tsp kaolin clay
1 tbsp cocoa powder, plus extra for colour-matching
¼ tsp ground cloves, plus extra for colour-matching
1 tsp ground cinnamon, plus extra for colour-matching
¼ tsp marula oil
5 drops frankincense essential oil

Put the arrowroot powder in a glass bowl and one by one add the remaining ingredients, stirring to fully combine between each addition. Once you have an even colour, test the colour on the back of your hand. If your skin tone is lighter, add a little more arrowroot; if it is darker, add a little more cocoa powder (you can play around with the clove and cinnamon, too, if it helps get the colour just right). Remember to go pinch by pinch until you get the perfect colour. Transfer the powder to an airtight cosmetics pot and use as necessary.

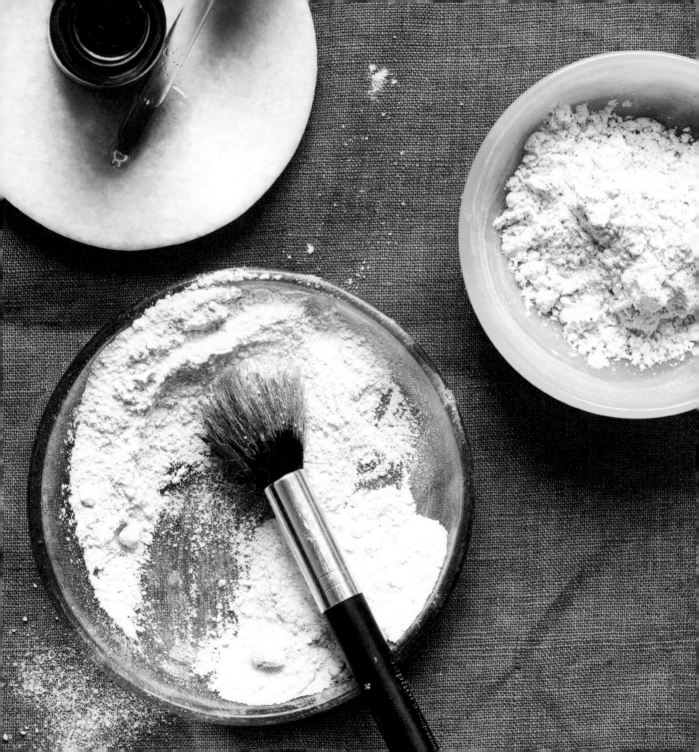

Marula Oil Bronzing Powder

There's nothing better than the day after you've been to the beach and your face has that beautiful, sun-kissed glow; it's gorgeous and it signifies health. I use a bronzer along my cheekbones to create that beach radiance all year round.

Makes about 15g/½oz
Shelf life: 6 months

1 tbsp zinc oxide
½ tsp gold mica, plus extra for colour-matching, as necessary
Brown and red iron oxides (individual amounts will vary according to colour, but you'll need about 5g/⅛oz altogether)
5 drops marula oil

Put the zinc oxide in a small, glass bowl and add the gold mica, stirring to combine. Mix in the brown and red oxides and add a little more gold mica if you feel the colour needs it, until you get just the colour you're looking for.

Once you're happy with the colour, add the marula oil (this will help with the stickability of the bronzer on your skin) and mix really well. Transfer to a cosmetics pot and use as needed.

TANNING
#fakethebake

'There is no such thing as a healthy tan, unless it's fake.'

I'm a huge advocate of spending time in the sun; even just 15 minutes is enough to rejuvenate you. Obviously, a sun-kissed complexion looks healthy, but also the body needs the sun's rays in order to manufacture vitamin D, and to my mind there's no greater help for stress or depression than the warm kiss you get from some scheduled sun time.

Baking for hours, however, is not good for you. We all know about skin cancer (melanoma), and there's also no faster way to age your skin prematurely than roasting yourself like a festive turkey. So what to do if you're looking for some summer glow? Simple – you fake the bake!

X

Tea & Cocoa Self-tanning Cream

Making your own fake tan has numerous benefits; the best perhaps is that there's no orange! (After all, as natural as this recipe is, there's no carrot in it – and you can't look like a carrot if there *is* no carrot, right?) Store-bought tanners are hugely pricey and loaded with nasties. My way you save money and keep your skin nurtured, as well as getting that gorgeous bronzed look.

Makes about 250ml/9fl oz/1 cup
Shelf life: 3 weeks

1–2 regular tea bags
120g/4½oz shea butter
70g/2½oz coconut oil
¼ tsp sweet almond oil
25g/1oz raw cocoa powder,
   plus extra for colour-matching,
   if necessary

First, make the tea. Place the tea bags in 60ml/2fl oz/¼ cup boiling water and allow to steep for 15–20 minutes (how many tea bags and how long you steep will determine how dark your self-tanning lotion will be). Remove and discard the tea bags and leave the tea to cool.

Meanwhile, make a double boiler by placing a glass bowl over a pan of simmering water. Allow the water to lap at the bowl, but not to flow over the edges of the pan. Add the shea butter, coconut oil and sweet almond oil and allow to melt. Once the butter and oil mixture has melted, give it a stir and remove the bowl from the heat (take care – it will be hot). Stir well to combine.

Leave the mixture to cool, then use a hand whisk to whip it to a creamy consistency. Little by little, add the cooled tea, whipping again between each addition. Once you've incorporated all the tea, add the raw cocoa powder, again little by little, this time stopping if you reach a colour that you think is deep enough. Whip between each addition until you're happy.

Transfer the mixture to an airtight cosmetics pot until needed. To use, apply to the skin in an even layer, rubbing it in until your skin feels gorgeously smooth. The pigment in the tea will begin to darken your skin slowly, giving you a naturally sunkissed look a few hours later.

Shimmer Powder Blush

This powder blush takes fewer than 60 seconds to make and it's my absolute favourite. I go for the purple–pink hue of beetroot to colour my blusher. If that's your preference, too, try making your own beetroot powder for the full, natural treatment: roast the roots for 4 hours to extract the moisture, then grind them up in a coffee grinder – easy!

Makes about 40g/1½oz
Shelf life: 6 months

1 tbsp cornflour (cornstarch)
1–2 tbsp red iron oxide powder
  (for a redder hue), hibiscus
  powder (for a red–purple), or
  beetroot powder (for purple–
  pink), plus extra if needed
Pinch of silver mica powder
  (optional)
½ tsp raw cocoa powder (optional)
2 drops orange leaf essential oil

In a glass bowl, combine the cornflour and your chosen coloured powder. You don't have to use all 2 tbsp of the colour – add little by little and if you reach a colour that you like, stop (bear in mind you may need to go darker in the mixture than you think – test a little on the back of your hand to see what it looks like on your skin). Stir in the mica powder (if using; this will give the blusher that lovely shimmer) and add a little raw cocoa powder, if you like, to take any sharp edges off the redness. Finally, add the orange leaf essential oil – not only is this good for your skin (it's toning and balancing), it will help to bind the blusher when you apply it and it smells delicious. Store the blusher in an airtight cosmetics pot and apply as you would any shop-bought version.

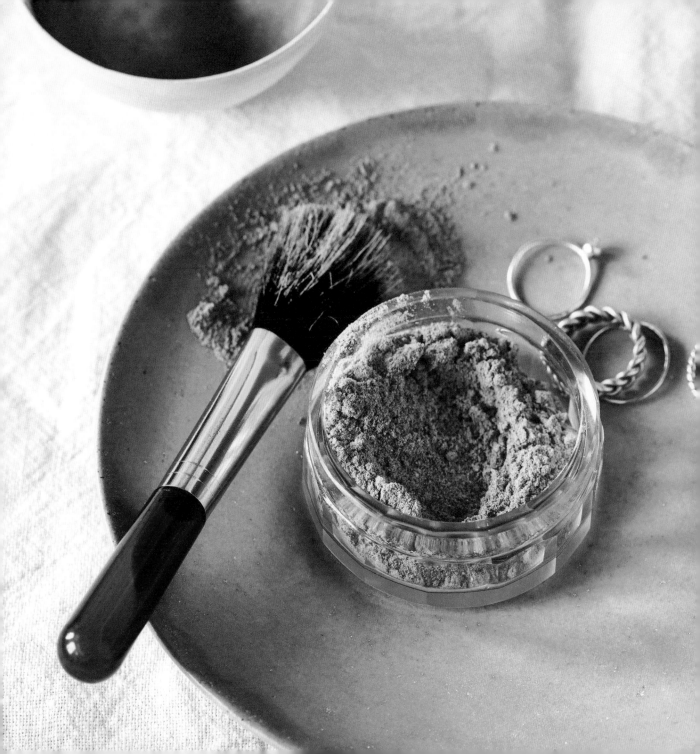

EYES
#eyeofthebeholder

There are a lot of guys who like nothing better than a girl who rolls out of bed, brushes her teeth, throws on a pair of jeans and a shirt and is ready for whatever life has to offer her (which is fortunate because I'm definitely one of those girls), but as the Bible tells us, there's a time for business and a time to relax. When I'm going out, I mean business and business (to me) is all about the eyes.

I've said that I'm lazy with makeup, but I'm not lazy when it comes to the windows to my soul; smoky eye-shadow, winged liner and full, thick lashes are my go-to essentials in the makeup department. There are a few reasons I love to fix my eyes, but there's something even more important to me than the windows themselves and that's what sits above them. Namely, my eyebrows. Back when I was losing all my hair, I also lost my eyebrows, which unfortunately never really grew back properly and I'll admit it makes me self-conscious. If I'm hitting the town, I can't leave the house without my eyebrows looking full and voluptuous (it sounds weird, but if you had half-missing brows you would understand my obsession), which makes DIY eyeliner gels and homemade mascaras – which double as brow pencils – the treasures in my makeup chest.

This section is all about the eye area. I've included my favourites to make and wear, and you'll never find my bathroom cabinet without them.

X

Defining Liquid Eyeliner

Eyeliner is so easy to make, it's madness to buy it ready made (the same goes for mascara; see opposite). I use this recipe all the time and it can double for mascara if you need to space-save while you travel (or you can use the mascara recipe as eyeliner, if you prefer). This also makes a great eyebrow filler.

Makes about 15ml/½fl oz/1 tbsp
Shelf life: 3 months

1 tsp aloe vera gel
½ tsp activated charcoal (for a
    black eyeliner) or raw cocoa
    powder (for brown)
½ tsp kaolin clay

Put the aloe vera gel in a small glass bowl and, pinch by pinch, add your chosen colourant. Stir to combine thoroughly, then add the kaolin clay and stir again. Transfer to a small cosmetics pot to store (I keep my eyeliner in a small glass container). To use, dab a little of the mixture on an eyeliner brush and apply neatly to your lid. Allow the first layer to dry and then repeat.

*You can use this formula to make any colour eyeliner you like – just use coloured mica rather than the charcoal or cocoa powder.

#everyonelovesaquickie A little activated charcoal mixed with a little coconut oil, dabbed on the end of a thin makeup brush and applied to your lids makes the perfect quickie eyeliner!

Long Lashes Mascara

I love that this mascara is as lash-lengthening as any shop-bought version I've tried. And if you want to add a bit of disco, use a coloured or sparkly mica, or even beetroot (purple), carmine (red) or spirulina (green) powder to make a mascara with a party hue. Try curling your lashes around the back of a teaspoon before you start (you can also use the stem to go for a winged-eyeliner look that would make Cleopatra proud).

Makes about 15ml/½fl oz/1 tbsp
Shelf life: 3 months

1 tsp aloe vera gel
¼ tsp extra-virgin olive oil
½ tsp activated charcoal
¼ tsp kaolin clay

In a bowl combine the aloe vera gel, extra-virgin olive oil, activated charcoal and kaolin clay until you have an even colour. Transfer to a small cosmetics pot to store (I pipe my mascara into an old mascara bottle). To use, dab a little mascara around all sides of a mascara brush and apply as you would a shop-bought product.

*If you don't have a mascara brush to hand, try using an old toothbrush to apply instead.

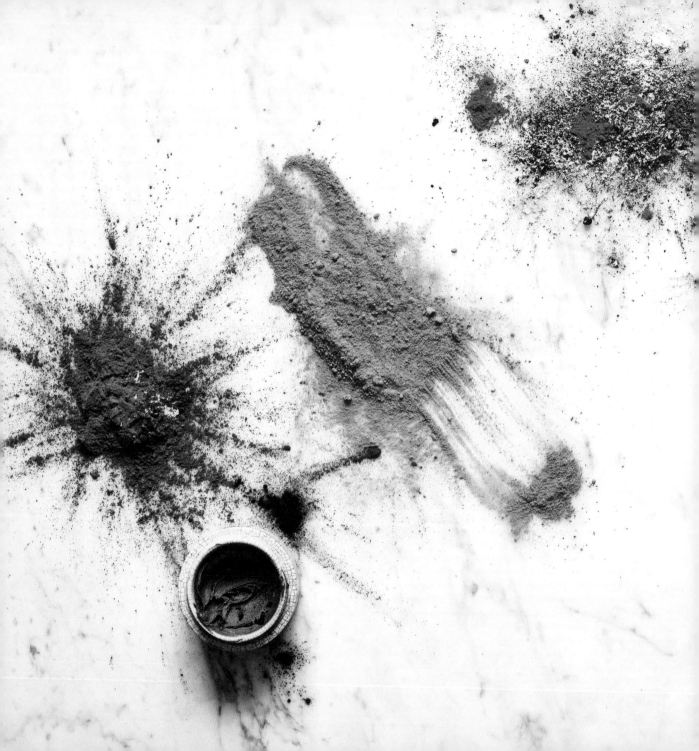

Colour-Me-Beautiful Eye Shadow

Makes about 15g/½oz
Shelf life: 3 months

½ tsp arrowroot powder
½ tsp silk mica
1 tsp colourant (see combinations
    in the box, below)
Pinch of silver mica (optional)
¼ tsp mango butter

On a night out (work or otherwise), I have several rituals to help me get into the right mental space and leave the house looking spiffy. First, I pick my outfit and matching accessories and then I choose my eye shadow; it might not seem like much, but the colour I choose for my eyes changes what makeup I'll wear on any other part of my face. It's a truth universally acknowledged that you should draw attention to one thing only – smoky eyes = pale lips; low-cut top = legs covered. Basically, less is more.

   Usually I'll go with a golden base on my eyes and use a little dark brown for contouring, but sometimes I like to get creative. In my cabinet I always have browns (in different shades) and a dark green on hand, but as this recipe takes all of 30 seconds to make, I can change my mind (and my colour) even when I have to be 'ready in five'. Use the colour combos below as a guide – feel free to mix-and-match until you get a colour that you love.

This brilliant eye shadow couldn't be easier. In a small, glass bowl, mix together the dry ingredients, including your chosen colour combo and the silver mica (it will give shimmer), if using, until you have an even colour. Add the mango butter and work it into the combined powders using the back of a spoon. When your eye shadow is perfectly even in colour, transfer to a small cosmetics pot to store. Apply using an eye shadow brush, just as you would a shop-bought product.

Natural Colour Combos

PASTEL PINK ¾ tsp hibiscus powder + ¼ tsp raw cocoa powder.

BARELY-THERE LAVENDER ½ tsp hibiscus powder + ¼ tsp ground nutmeg + ¼ tsp cocoa powder.

GRASS GREEN 1 tsp spirulina.

DEEP BLUE ¾ tsp blue iron oxide + ¼ tsp cocoa powder.

SMOKY BLUE ¾ tsp blue oxide + ¼ tsp activated charcoal.

PALE BROWN 1 tsp cocoa powder.

GOLDEN BROWN ¾ tsp ground turmeric + ¼ tsp ground nutmeg.

DARK BROWN ¾ tsp cocoa powder + ¼ tsp activated charcoal.

LIPS
#kissmequick

Possibly the most familiar and loved makeup product, lipstick was actually created to give the appearance of sexual excitement (the flush you get when aroused); these days, however, it's more about fashion than the 'come-to-bed-with-me' look.

I love a good lippy (usually red) and I use it to complete my outfit, much like an accessory. My lipstick can and does serve a purpose, but it's not the only thing that works up a kissable pout – there's also gloss and balm.

This section has something for everyone – whatever you like to use on your lips, with these recipes you'll always be ready for a first (or second) kiss.

X

Kissable Natural Lipstick

This recipe provides the base for making lipsticks and you can add whatever colours, herbs, spices and essential oils you like to give that gorgeous look and even flavour! The recipe takes about 5 minutes to make and another 5–10 minutes to set (depending on the room temperature). I like to add 1 tsp red oxide for my favourite red lippy with ½ tsp cinnamon to give a light glossy shimmer. Sometimes, though, I go for shimmer alone.

Makes 1 tube of lipstick
Shelf life: 6 months

5g/⅛oz beeswax
5g/⅛oz shea butter or mango butter
5g/⅛oz coconut oil
Colourant of choice, such as:
    2 tsp red iron oxide (for red);
    1 tsp ground cinnamon (for tan and shimmer); 1 tsp beetroot powder (for pink)
2 drops skin-healthy essential oil, such as strawberry seed, spearmint or cucumber seed (optional)

Make a double boiler by placing a glass bowl over a pan of simmering water. Allow the water to lap at the bowl, but not to flow over the edges of the pan. Add the wax, butter and coconut oil and allow to melt. Once the butter and oil mixture has melted, give it a stir and remove the bowl from the heat (take care – it will be hot). Stir well to combine. Add your chosen colourant and stir again until you have an even hue; then stir through the essential oil (if using). Keep stirring until the wax is just starting to cool a little and very slightly thicken up, then quickly pour it through a funnel into an old lipstick or lip balm tube. Leave to set at room temperature, about 5–10 minutes. To use, apply straight from the stick, as appropriate.

*You can buy packaging for lipsticks and makeup online (see Directory, page 124).

*Practice makes perfect with this – you'll need to work quickly to get the mixture into the tube while it's still pourable but holding its colour evenly. Don't give up! The results are so worth it.

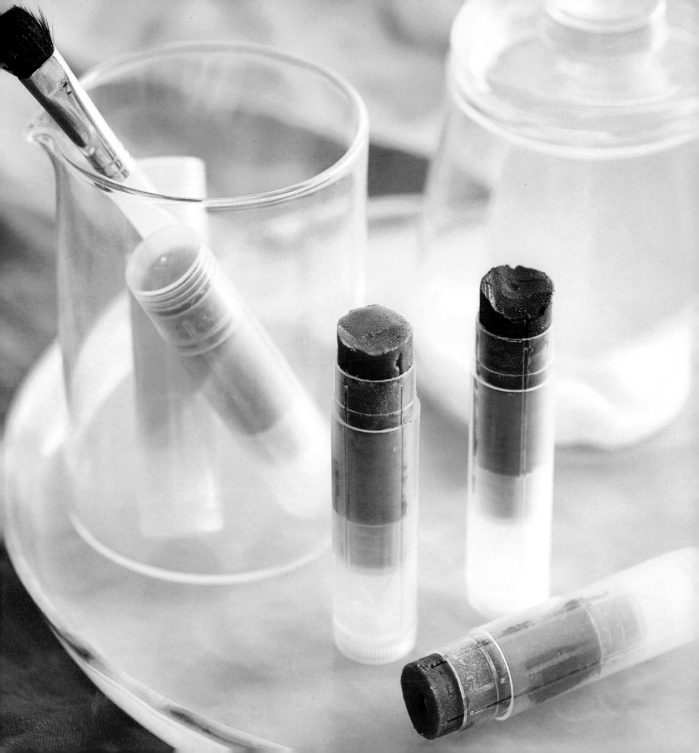

Conditioning Lip Gloss

This gloss is a base: you can use it plain as a lip conditioner (I do this when my lips are feeling dry) or you can add colour. If you do want to add colour, mix in just ½ tsp at a time until you're happy. If things go too dark, add a little arrowroot powder to lighten. The essential oils I've suggested are all good choices for moisturizing dry lips.

Makes about 75g/2½oz
Shelf life: 6 months

2 tbsp castor oil
1 tbsp sweet almond oil
10g/¼oz coconut oil
1 tsp macadamia nut or apricot
 kernel oil
½ tsp walnut oil
5g/⅛oz beeswax
1 tsp vegetable glycerine
5 drops skin-healthy essential
 oil, such as strawberry seed,
 spearmint or coriander seed
 (optional)

Make a double boiler by placing a glass bowl over a pan of simmering water. Allow the water to lap at the bowl, but not to flow over the edges of the pan. Add the castor oil, nut oils and wax and allow to melt. Once the oils and wax have melted, give them a stir to combine and remove the bowl from the heat (take care – it will be hot). Stir well again.

Allow the oil and wax mixture to cool, then pop it in the fridge for 10–15 minutes. Remove the cooled mixture from the fridge and use a hand blender to whip it up so that you get a lovely, creamy consistency. Add the vegetable glycerine and whip again. Finally, stir in the essential oils (if using), then transfer to a small cosmetics pot and allow to set.

To use, apply with a lipstick brush or your finger. The castor oil in the mixture should give you a gorgeous glossy shine.

Healing Chia Lip Gloss

Makes about 75g/2½oz
Shelf life: 6 months

2 tbsp castor oil
1 tbsp sweet almond oil
10g/¼oz coconut oil
1 tsp macadamia nut oil
½ tsp walnut oil
5g/⅛oz beeswax
1 tsp vegetable glycerine
½ tsp raw honey
1 tsp chia seed oil

Bursting with essential fatty acids, vitamins and antioxidants, chia seed oil has the wonderful ability to deeply nourish and balance all skin types.

I discovered the benefits when my lips were suffering during a winter fashion shoot. In fashion it's very common to shoot summer garments in the middle of winter and vice versa. Standing in a light dress when it's freezing cold or in a huge coat when it's sweltering is not my idea of fun, and it also wreaks havoc on your skin. When it comes to the lips, topsy-turvy seasonal dressing can quickly dry them out and make them chapped. Between photo-calls and catwalks, to ensure I keep my work pout, I apply just a little chia seed oil diluted in sweet almond oil every 10 minutes (then I just reapply the necessary lippy on top).

Once I started making my own cosmetics, that simple remedy became the inspiration for something more substantial, but equally healing. So, here it is: the ultimate lip-relief gloss.

Make a double boiler by placing a glass bowl over a pan of simmering water. Allow the water to lap at the bowl, but not to flow over the edges of the pan. Add the castor oil, nut oils and wax and allow to melt. Once the oils and wax have melted, give them a stir to combine and remove the bowl from the heat (take care – it will be hot). Stir well again.

Allow the oil and wax mixture to cool, then pop it in the fridge until it is soft set (keep an eye on it – when it's opaque and just starting to solidify, it's ready). Remove the cooled mixture from the fridge and use a hand blender to whip it up so that you get a lovely, creamy consistency. Add the vegetable glycerine and honey and whip again. Finally, whip in the chia seed oil. Transfer to a small cosmetics pot and allow to set completely.

To use, apply with a lipstick brush or the tip of your finger.

Partytime Lip Gloss

As I'm sure you can tell by now, I love red lips! This lip gloss puts passion in your pout and tells the world you're ready to party! I've given the options of ground freeze-dried raspberries for a bright, pinky-red colour or red oxide for a russet red – adding a little blue will take the edge off either, if you prefer. Whatever you choose, this is a gloss that says lips are a serious business.

Makes about 75g/2½oz
Shelf life: 6 months

2 tbsp castor oil
1 tbsp sweet almond oil
10g/¼oz coconut oil
1 tsp macadamia nut oil
½ tsp walnut oil
7g beeswax
1 tsp vegetable glycerine
1 tsp ground freeze-dried
   raspberries (for party pink)
   or red iron oxide powder (for
   sultry rusty red)
Pinch of blue mica or natural
   indigo powder (optional)

Make a double boiler by placing a glass bowl over a pan of simmering water. Allow the water to lap at the bowl, but not to flow over the edges of the pan. Add the castor oil, nut oils and wax and allow to melt. Once the oils and wax have melted, give them a stir to combine and remove the bowl from the heat (take care – it will be hot). Stir well again.

Allow the oil and wax mixture to cool, then pop it in the fridge until it is just soft set (keep an eye on it – when it's opaque and starting to solidify, it's ready). Remove the cooled mixture from the fridge and use a hand blender to whip it up so that you get a lovely, creamy consistency. Add the vegetable glycerine and whip again. Finally, stir in the red colourant and the blue mica or natural indigo powder (if using), then transfer to a small cosmetics pot and allow to set. To use, apply with a lipstick brush or the tip of your finger.

#everyonelovesaquickie Next time you're making roasted beetroot (try them – they're delicious), rub a slice around your mouth for colour and then cover with a little coconut oil to set. You can also do this with cherries for a red colour and pomegranates for a light pink shade.

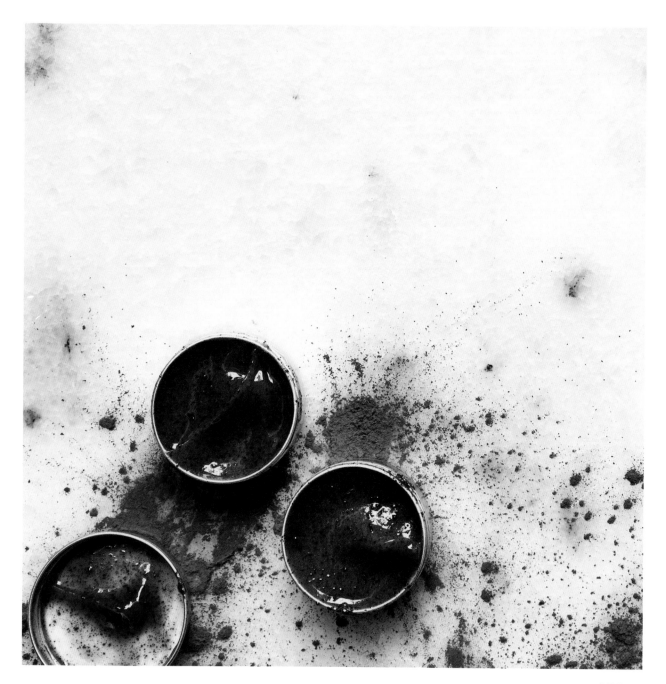

Pearly Sheen Lip Balm

Lip balms are all about hydrating and nourishing your lips, but that doesn't mean they have to be plain and boring. This recipe adds a little sheen of excitement to your pout.

Makes about 50g/2oz
Shelf life: 6 months

2 tsp apricot kernel oil
10g/¼oz coconut oil
5g/⅛oz beeswax
10g/¼oz mango butter
½ tsp aloe vera gel
½ tsp vitamin E oil
2 drops tea tree essential oil
½ tsp hibiscus powder
Large pinch of ground cinnamon
½–1 tsp shimmer pearl mica
   powder

Make a double boiler by placing a glass bowl over a pan of simmering water. Allow the water to lap at the bowl, but not to flow over the edges of the pan. Add the apricot kernel oil, coconut oil, wax, and mango butter and allow to melt. Remove the bowl from the pan (take care – the bowl will be hot) and add the aloe vera, vitamin E oil and tea tree essential oil. Leave the mixture to cool until it is opaque and soft set, then use a hand whisk to whip it up to a creamy consistency.

Add the hibiscus powder, ground cinnamon and shimmer pearl mica (you can add the mica powder little by little if you want to test the shimmer as you go). Whisk again until you have a completely even colour and sheen through the balm. Transfer to a lip-balm jar (you may need more than one, depending upon the size) and leave for about 10–20 minutes to set. Store at room temperature. To use, apply with the tip of your finger.

Golden Glow Lip Balm

Think of this as a bronzer for your lips to give your pout a little sun-kissed, 'I've-just-come-back-from-the-Islands' glow.

Makes about 50g/2oz
Shelf life: 6 months

2 tsp apricot kernel oil
10g/¼oz coconut oil
5g/⅛oz beeswax
10g/¼oz mango butter
½ tsp aloe vera gel
½ tsp vitamin E oil
2 drops orange leaf essential oil
¼ tsp ground cinnamon
½ tsp gold mica powder

Make a double boiler by placing a glass bowl over a pan of simmering water. Allow the water to lap at the bowl, but not to flow over the edges of the pan. Add the apricot kernel oil, coconut oil, wax, and mango butter and allow to melt. Remove the bowl from the pan (take care – the bowl will be hot). Allow the mixture to cool until it is opaque and soft set, then use a hand whisk to whip it to a creamy consistency.

Add the aloe vera, vitamin E oil and orange leaf essential oil. Whip again, then add the cinnamon and gold mica powder. Whip again until you have a completely even colour and sheen through the balm. Transfer to a lip-balm jar (you may need more than one, depending upon the size) and leave for about 10–20 minutes to set. Store at room temperature. To use, apply with the tip of your finger.

NAILS
#atyourfingertips

Most conventional nail polishes (that is, those mostly found on store shelves) offer up a noxious ingredient list of substances, including the 'toxic trio' of formaldehyde, toluene and dibutyl phthalate (DBP; see page 10).

I'm always having nail polish applied and reapplied to my fingers and toes and, as pretty as it looks at the time, what's happening beneath are nails that are becoming stained and brittle – basically, in terrible condition.

Making your own nail polish is tough (honestly – it's for hardcore, seasoned DIY-ers only) and – I admit – it's one thing that's easier just to buy. If you're not that hardcore yet (I hear you!), the best store-bought nail polish is water-based and you can buy it online made by these brands:

Honeybee Gardens
Aquarella
Scotch Naturals
Piggy Paint

For the times inbetween, I'm offering up a gorgeous nail conditioner that will leave a soft sheen on your nails that is perfect for every day. And for the times when you do use nail polish, check out the #everyonelovesaquickie acetone-free removers to minimize the harsh effects.

X

Nail Conditioning Oil

Makes about 60ml/2fl oz/¼ cup
Shelf life: 6 weeks

½ tsp beeswax, or candelilla
  or soy wax
3 tbsp grapeseed oil
1 tbsp vitamin E oil
½ tsp jojoba oil
2 drops lavender essential oil
1 drop frankincense essential oil

Often it feels like I've been experimenting for a thousand years trying to come up with the perfect formula for a homemade nail polish and still the solution eludes me! Instead, I use this gorgeous nail-conditioning oil, which leaves my nails with a soft sheen. The essential oils will help to strengthen the keratin in your nails, making them strong as well as supple.

Make a double boiler by placing a small glass bowl over a pan of simmering water. Allow the water to lap at the bowl, but not to flow over the edges of the pan. Add the wax, grapeseed oil and vitamin E oil and allow to warm and mingle as the wax melts. Once everything is combined, remove the bowl from the pan (take care – the bowl will be hot) and allow the mixture to cool slightly, then add the jojoba oil and essential oils and stir again. Transfer the mixture to an empty nail varnish bottle. To use, put a few drops of the oil on a cotton bud and apply to your nails one by one, re-soaking the cotton bud as necessary.

Acetone-free Nail Polish Removers
#everyonelovesaquickie

VINEGAR & LEMON
Use 2 parts white wine vinegar with 1 part lemon juice. Soak your nails in hot water for 10–15 minutes, then dip a cotton-wool pad in the vinegar mixture and rub away the polish.

GIN OR VODKA
Soak your nails in a bowl of gin or vodka for 10–15 minutes, then use a cotton-wool pad (or an old toothbrush for really stubborn bits) to rub the polish away.

TOOTHPASTE & BICARB
Mix 1 tbsp toothpaste with 1 tsp bicarbonate of soda (baking soda), then use a nailbrush to scrub away the polish.

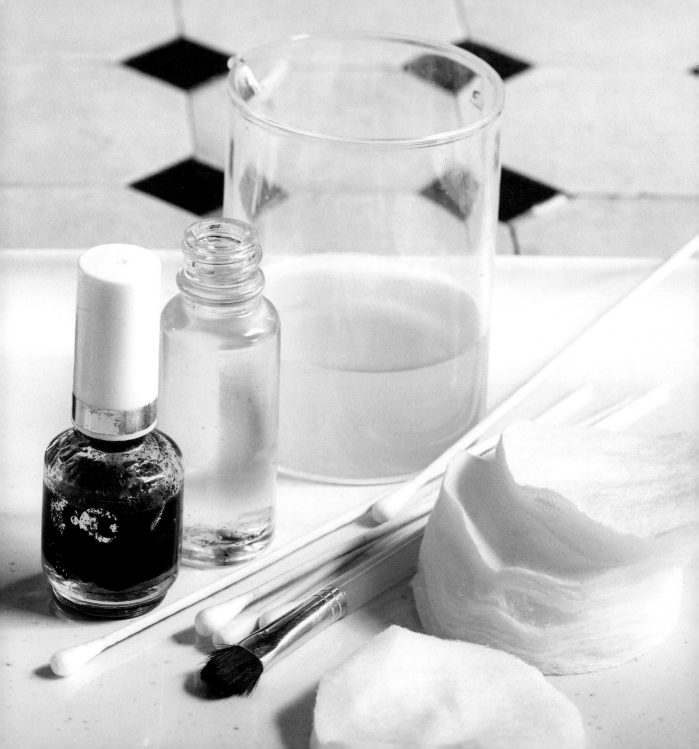

FRAGRANCE
#arosebyanyothername

'What do I wear to bed? Chanel no.5 of course.'
Marilyn Monroe

The thing about perfume is that it all comes down to the essential oils –
we have been using them to make scents to mask our body odour for hundreds
of years... certainly long before anyone dreamt up the idea of adding any of the
chemical nasties that appear in so many modern-day fragrances. Take note: the
perfume industry isn't like the food industry – perfume manufacturers are not presently
under any obligation to tell you what they use to make those bottles of liquid scent
smell so good. So, let's get back to basics. If essential oils is where it began, then
essential oils is where I'm going: straight to nature, in combinations that I can
mix-and-match to personalize a perfume just for me.

Marilyn Monroe may have worn Chanel no.5; I'm wearing Alex no.1.

X

Spiced Jasmine Perfume

Makes about 125ml/4fl oz/½ cup
Shelf life: 6 months

125ml/4fl oz/½ cup mild carrier
   oil (see list below) – I like sweet
   almond oil for this blend
10 drops mandarin essential oil
10 drops vanilla essential oil
5 drops jasmine essential oil
5 drops rose geranium essential oil
5 drops coriander seed essential
   oil
½ tbsp vodka

Mild carrier oils – choose from:
Sweet almond oil
Jojoba oil
Apricot kernel oil
Sunflower oil
Safflower oil
Macadamia nut oil
Kukui nut oil
Avocado oil

We spend staggering amounts of money every year on bottled perfumes. It's madness given that perfume is basically just blended essential oils. So, if it's that simple – why not make it yourself? Here is my favourite homemade blend. I love it because its floral and citrus scent is so personal to me, each element reminding me of something or someone special. Feel free to experiment with your own favourite scents, just remember to dilute the essential oils in the same proportions with the carrier oil, and choose essential oils that are non-sensitizing for your skin.

Pour the carrier oil into a small glass bowl and add your essential oils 1 or 2 drops at a time, stirring between each addition. Don't be afraid to add more or less according to your preference – jasmine essential oil, for example, has a particularly strong scent, so you may need fewer than 5 drops (or you may love it so much you want to add more). Give the blend a stir and a sniff at every stage until you're happy. Then, add the vodka and stir to fully combine (the alcohol will help the perfume 'dry' on your skin, rather than feeling oily).

Transfer the finished blend to a dark-coloured glass cosmetics bottle, which will protect the oils from degrading in the light, preserving their scents and properties. Store in a cool, dark place. To use, dab a little of the blend on your wrists, just as you would shop-bought perfume.

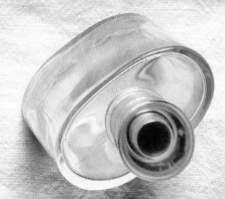

Directory

Organic Supermarkets & Online Suppliers

Amazon (worldwide) www.amazon.com
Health Emporium, The (AU) www.healthemporium.com.au
Mr Vitamins (AU) www.mrvitamins.com.au
Planet Organic (UK) www.planetorganic.com
Westerly Natural Market (USA) www.westerlynaturalmarket.com
Wholefoods Market (UK/USA/Canada) www.wholefoodsmarket.com

Cosmetic Ingredient Suppliers

From Nature with Love (USA) www.fromnaturewithlove.com
Holland & Barrett (UK) www.hollandandbarrett.com
Mountain Rose Herbs (USA) www.mountainroseherbs.com
New Directions (AU) www.newdirections.com.au
New Directions Aromatics (UK) www.newdirectionsuk.com
Nikita Naturals (AU) www.nikitanaturals.com
Skin Essential Actives (ASIA) www.skinessentialactives.com

Bottles & Packaging Suppliers

All In Packaging (UK) www.allinpackaging.co.uk
Escentials of Australia (AU) www.escentialsofaustralia.com
Just Jars (AU) www.justjars.com.au
SKS Bottles (USA) www.sks-bottle.com
World of Bottles (UK) www.world-of-bottles.co.uk

Worldwide Natural Beauty Suppliers

The Model Handmade www.themodelhandmade.com
100% Pure www.100percentpure.com
Lush www.lush.com.au
Morrocco Method www.morroccomethod.com

Acknowledgements

A huge thank you to my incredible family and friends, without whom this book would never have been written.

To my mum, for your never ending wisdom and for making so many of these recipes with me (even though you hate cooking).

My soul mate, life guru and sister, Stephanie, for testing each and every one of my creations so diligently and for encouraging me to put my scribbled bits of paper into a book.

To my little Yorkie, Rosie, who reminds me every day that animals are to be loved and never test-subjects.

To Harley, thank you for teaching me what it means to be happy. All of this is all I have and all I have is yours.

To all the men and women who love and are learning to love themselves; may you be inspired and guided to nurture the most valuable asset you have – YOU!

And to my son, for inspiring and guiding me on this path; I am eternally grateful. We had a lifetime together in the space of a single moment and I will love you all the days of my life.

Index

#everyonelovesaquickie

Here's a handy reference guide for all you quickie fans!

Blemish busters 68
Cleansers 32
Eyeliner 104
Face masks 84
Face scrubs 76
Foaming dispenser 24
Foundation 91
Lip gloss 114
Moisturizers 52
Nail polish remover 120
Serums 62
Toners 42

PUBLISHER'S NOTES

Bentonite clay is used in several recipes in this book. Bentonite is a positively charged element which means it attaches to negative elements. It cannot come into contact with anything metallic or it becomes toxic. Recipes using bentonite must be made with wooden or plastic utensils.

Essential oils can be potent. Always read the labels before using, check for contraindications and ensure safe dilutions in a base oil or soap.

Neither the author nor the publisher can take any responsibility for any illness or injury caused as a result of following any of the advice or using any of the recipes or methods contained in this book.

PUBLISHER'S ACKNOWLEDGEMENTS

With thanks to photographer Rachel Whiting, and to stylist and home economist Aya Nishimura.

First published in the United Kingdom in 2017 by
Pavilion
43 Great Ormond Street
London
WC1N 3HZ

Copyright © Pavilion Books Group Ltd 2017
Text copyright © Alex Brennan 2017

ISBN 978-1-91121-689-6

A CIP catalogue record for this book is available from the British Library.

10 9 8 7 6 5 4 3 2 1

The information and material provided in this publication is representative of the author's opinions and views. The information and material is presented in good faith; however, no warranty is given, nor are results guaranteed. Pavilion does not have any control over, or any responsibility for, any author or third party websites referred to in this book.

Reproduction by Mission Productions Ltd, Hong Kong
Printed and bound by 1010 Printing International Ltd, China

This book can be ordered direct from the publisher at www.pavilionbooks.com